BRAIN STORMS

RECOVERY FROM
TRAUMATIC BRAIN INJURY

by
JOHN W. CASSIDY, M.D.

This book is not intended to replace personal medical care and/or professional supervision; there is no substitute for the experience and information that your doctor or mental health professional can provide. Rather, it is our hope that this book will provide additional information to help people understand the nature of traumatic brain injury and its effects on its victims and their families.

Proper treatment should always be tailored to the individual. If you read something in this book that seems to conflict with your doctor or mental health professional's instructions, contact him/her. There may be sound reasons for recommending treatment that may differ from the information presented in this book.

If you have any questions about any treatment in this book, please consult your doctor or mental health care professional.

In addition, the names and cases used in this book do not represent actual people, but are composite cases drawn from several sources.

The Neurobehavioral Institute of Houston

The Neurobehavioral Institute of Houston is a free-standing medical specialty hospital treating patients who show significant behavioral, cognitive or emotional problems as a result of brain injury/illness. Individualized programs integrate strategies from neurology, psychiatry, physical medicine and rehabilitation with adult, adolescent and children's programs. Community homes and apartment living are available for longer term treatment or supported living.

ACKNOWLEDGMENTS

The author wishes to acknowledge the invaluable assistance of Karla Dougherty without whom this book would never have been written and Margaret Preston who saw to it that once it was written it was finally completed.

DEDICATION

This book is dedicated to MALC, LLFC, ELC, RJC, and SHF.

CONTENTS

About the Author

John W. Cassidy, M.D. is the Medical Director of the
Neurobehavioral Institute of Houston, a medical specialty
hospital designed for the care and treatment of patients
with neuromedical and neurobehavioral difficulties. Having trained through the Harvard Teaching Hospital System
and McLean Hospital, Dr. Cassidy has ten years of extensive experience in his field. He is a recognized leader in the
field of neuropsychiatry and has published a number of
papers on a wide range of psychiatric topics with a special
interest in psychopharmacologic treatments and their selective implementation in the rehabilitation of brain-injured
patients. He is a member of the National Head Injury
Foundation and serves on its Psychiatric Advisory Commit-
tee as well as the Advisory Council to the Texas Head
Injury Association.

THE SILENT EPIDEMIC

I hope that:

- I can have a job that I enjoy.
- I can get a driver's license.
- I can help my daughter and my family.
- I can be independent.

Simple wishes. Simple dreams. This list of personal goals could come from almost anyone—and, under normal circumstances, be within grasp. But this list was not written down one evening amidst the papers and bills on a cluttered desk. It wasn't scrawled on a notepad next to a kitchen phone. These aspirations weren't resolutions thought up after a New Year's Eve celebration. This list of personal goals came from Peter Stevens*, a patient at the Neuro-behavioral Institute of Houston, a man whose traumatic brain injury had brought him to program after program for over ten years, an intelligent, hard-working man whose accident turned him into a troubled, impulsive, often depressed human being, who, two weeks after his accident, couldn't even recall his name—let alone write down a list of personal goals. But now, through effective rehabilitation, Peter Stevens can not only write and remember what he's written, but begin to see his list of personal goals come true.

---

*Patient names, and their identifying characteristics, have been changed to protect patient privacy.

THE SILENT EPIDEMIC

Peter Stevens is not an isolated case. Thanks to advances in emergency medical care, diagnostic technology, and medical research and rehabilitation, more and more people are surviving tragic accidents that once would have claimed their lives. Bodies can be nurtured and healed, measures can be taken to prevent pain, death rates have declined. But the lives of these survivors of traumatic brain injury (TBI) have often been irrevocably changed.

Unfortunately, survival does not always mean recovery—especially when it comes to the brain. From the way a person falls in a bicycle spill to vital oxygen loss during a heart attack, injury to the brain is an ever-present danger. Yes, there are less fatalities—but we are seeing more and more of the complications of brain injury when the individual has seemingly been rehabilitated and returned home.

The fact is that traumatic brain injury is more common than you might think. There are 500,000 cases a year in America and 200,000 of these are serious enough to require hospitalization. Indeed, TBI has already been labeled "The Silent Epidemic."

Some statistics:

• TBI is nearly three times more common in men than women. Why? Because males, especially in their youth, take more risks than their female counterparts. From fast cars and motorcycles to substance and alcohol abuse, young men are traditionally more prone to "wild" behavior. Men have also traditionally been drawn to careers that involve some danger: construction work, flying airplanes and service in the armed forces.

• The two most vulnerable age groups for TBI-associated deaths are youths aged 15 to 24 (with 77 percent of the fatalities the result of motor vehicle accidents) and senior citizens aged 75 and older (with falls being the number one cause in 43 percent of reported cases).

• Ten percent of all brain injuries come from sports—especially football, baseball, and basketball.

• Approximately 1,300 people die from head injury caused by bicycle accidents every year.

• Falls are the third leading cause of death in children aged one to four.

• TBI costs society over $4 billion a year, including emergency medical treatment, rehabilitation services, and loss of income.

• Alcohol and substance abuse can cause accidents—which can lead to brain injury. Today, less people drink and drive—with the result that from 1982–87 deaths due to drunken driving were reduced by 6,400.

• Unfortunately, brain injury that goes undetected and untreated can lead to a host of neurobehavioral difficulties, like anxiety and depression. Also, a brain injured victim can become so depressed and frightened over his injury that he will turn to alcohol or drugs in order to cope.

• A study of 160 brain injured children in a pediatric brain rehabilitation center showed that early intervention directly influenced outcome: the earlier a child was brought to the center, the better his chances of improvement.

WHAT IS TBI?

Although there are risk factors that make its occurrence more likely, TBI is not preordained. It is not cast in stone. It can happen to anyone, a result of a tragic accident that can occur in the blink of an eye—changing the life of the person who survives it and his or her family forever.

Like cancer and other tragedies, no one wants to know about TBI until it happens to someone they know and love. This makes sense. Unpleasant subjects are only sought out when we see them used as entertainment in tv's soaps, in movies, or in our sweeping, saga meganovels. But, as we have seen, TBI is an unfortunate fact of modern life and, if someone you care about is suffering from one, you need to know as much as possible to set the right kind of help into motion—fast.

Not only does early rehabilitation affect a person's ultimate outcome, but it can help both you and your loved ones cope with a suddenly strange and difficult world. Because it is the brain that is injured, the symptoms you will see will be very different than those your spouse or child would show if he or she had broken a leg or came down with the flu.

He might forget what he just said—or what you just said to him. She might not remember what she set out to do this morning. He might become irritable, throwing things and threatening people. She might become depressed and anxious. He might suffer from insomnia. She might become incontinent and incapable of keeping herself groomed. He might not acknowledge the left side of his body—eating food on only one side of his plate, putting only one arm through a shirt. She might have her thoughts frozen in time, believing she is still a teenager—although, in reality, her hair is grey and she's a grandmother in her late sixties.

In short, symptoms of traumatic brain injury vary from individual to individual. They are as unique as the personality of the person suffering its outrageous fortune. But, although symptoms range from the mildly idiosyncratic to the extremely painful, they tend to fall into three main categories:

- Impaired cognitive functioning
- Behavioral and emotional changes
- Physical handicaps

These three categories together create the most troubling symptom of TBI of all...

THE ALIEN SELF

There is no greater nightmare than waking up and discovering that the self we took for granted is gone. From *1984* to *The Invasion of the Body Snatchers,* the loss of self has been the theme behind many a classic and best-selling science-fiction fantasy. But what makes TBI even more insidious is the fact that its victims don't realize that they are different—but you, their parent, their spouse, their friend or lover, know beyond a shadow of a doubt. Both of you are joined together in extremely unusual and complex pain. Together, you must make the difficult journey back—to a functioning family, to fulfilling friendships and to productive activity that are the hallmarks of successful rehabilitation.

It is rediscovering those things we take for granted, those very things that make us human that led me into the burgeoning field of neuropsychiatry, combining my knowledge of neurology and psychiatry to help people cope with the consequences of their head injury and once again become contributing members of society.

To this end, I have written this book, taking you first through the landscape of the brain where you will learn the basics of how it functions—as well as discover the different kind of problems that occur when it is injured. Then, and most importantly, I will take you step-by-step through rehabilitation. Based on my experiences as the Medical Director of the Neurobehavioral Institute of Houston, the rehabilitation program you will read about is based not only on an understanding of the brain, but on the indefinable individuality of each patient as well, on their personal struggle to "refind" themselves: a task that is a TBI victim's greatest challenge.

At our journey's end, you will not only have a working knowledge of how a person suffering from TBI can be helped—but you, yourself, will be better equipped to accept, appreciate, and more peacefully live with this changed person.

I believe there is a rich and varied life after traumatic brain injury. After reading *Brain Storms: Recovery from Traumatic Brain Injury*, it is my great hope that you will too.

Let's begin . . . .

PART I

BRAIN MATTERS

ONE

HOW THE BRAIN WORKS

"The human brain is simply the most marvelous organ in the known universe."

—Dr. Miles Herkenham, NIMH neuroscientist

When Dr. P. first came to see the renowned neurologist Oliver Sacks, he seemed perfectly sound. He was an affable, intelligent professor with a gift for music. Yet something was amiss. On occasion, Dr. P. would be unable to recognize a familiar face—or he'd imagine a person standing before him when, in reality, what stood in his way was a banister knob or a fire hydrant. He and his wife didn't seek out help at first; the incidents were dismissed as minor and funny. Besides, Dr. P. was still a distinguished member of his faculty at his music school. But things did not improve. Eventually, they came to see Dr. Sacks.

The examination proved futile—until Dr. Sacks told Dr. P. that he could put his shoe back on. Dr. P. couldn't understand what Dr. Sacks was talking about—or what the leather-soled object in his hand was. And, when he rose to leave the office, he literally tried to lift off his wife's head—an incident that became the title story of Oliver Sacks's book, *The Man Who Mistook His Wife for a Hat.*

Ultimately, Dr. P. was found to have a brain tumor. But it was not until his mind began to deteriorate that his problem was noted and help was sought.

And why would Dr. P. have contacted a doctor? The fact is that when things are running smoothly, we rarely question them. We don't give it a thought that, say, the refrigerator is keeping food cold or that the roof over our heads is intact.

Similarly, although we might have periodic checkups, we don't run to a doctor because we're feeling great. This is especially true when it comes to our brains. When the brain is functioning the way it should, we don't step back and think about how well "it" enables us to hear a symphony, how confidently "it" knows we need sleep, how perfect "its" ability to set the appropriate emotional tone.

But think of how extraordinary these "normal" brain functions are. From maintaining blood pressure to swallowing food, from the exultation of holding a loved one to the confusing pain of loss, from following a recipe to dialing a phone—what an extraordinary, amazing, and miraculous organ the "normal" brain is!

GRAY MATTER

A simple truth: the brain is the organ of the mind. And damage to our brain will affect our minds—our behavior, our emotions, our personality, and our cognitive abilities. But in order to determine what's wrong when a brain is injured, we need to know what's right when it's working properly. We need to know the "normal" functions of the different parts of the brain, and how these different parts "speak" to each other to create action, emotion, and thought:

1. The Ancient Brainstem

When we touch a hot stove, the nerve endings in our fingers carry the message *hot-pain* to the spinal cord—which, along with the brain, makes up the central nervous system (CNS). The spinal cord carries *hot-pain* up to the brainstem, or more specifically, the *medulla,* its first stop.

No, it isn't a beast from Greek mythology. The inch-long medulla handles all those automatic functions that keep us alive: breathing, swallowing, blood pressure regulation, and more. You'll also find controls for every sense except sight and smell. (These go directly to higher parts of the brain without stopping—which explains why these senses are always felt more acutely, why a certain scent or flash of vision can bring back a powerful rush of memory.) The medulla is always on the alert, ready to retrieve messages like *hot-pain* and relay them to other areas of the brain for deciphering and action.

The next landmark is the *pons,* which means, quite literally, the "bridge," because it links the lower regions of the brain with its higher, more evolved areas.

Passing through the pons, *hot-pain* leaves the "outskirts" of the central nervous system and begins to enter the suburbs of the more sophisticated cities of the brain's upper regions. But instead of malls and main streets, you'll find the *midbrain,* which integrates rudimentary sight and sound.

The entire brainstem looks very much like a reptile's complete brain—which is why it is sometimes called the reptilian brain. The next time you wonder why snakes can't add two plus two, you'll know it's because their brains stop here.

BRAIN STORMING

Brain Statistics

- The whole brain weighs less than three pounds— but it can store more information than all the libraries in the entire world!
- There are between 10 and 100 *billion* neurons in the basic brain.
- By the time we are seven years old, our brain is almost adult in weight and size. There will be no more neurons, no more growth. But a rich, stimulating environment will increase the number of synapses between cells.
- An irony: When we live, we learn how to do more and more with less and less.

---

2. The Cerebellum Two-Step

It stands for "little brain" and it's attached to the back of the brainstem. This "little brain" is not that small when you consider it coordinates all our movements, modulating, maintaining, and adjusting our every step, our every stance. Recent studies have also discovered that the cerebellum stores some of our simple learned responses—everything from singing "Happy Birthday" to clasping an extended hand.

3. The Diencephalon Duo

All roads in the brainstem lead to the *diencephalon*. Located just above the midbrain, this area of the brain contains the thalamus and the hypothalamus—the two all-important gateways to higher thought, emotion, and mental health.

Every bit of information, every message from the insignificant to the sublime, goes through the thalamus—a customs clerk of sorts who does a preliminary classification search before delineating what part of the brain gets what message.

Right below the thalamus is the hypothalamus, the brain's control tower. It is a dynamo of function, regulating our:

- eating patterns
- sleeping and waking cycles
- body temperature
- chemical balances
- emotional tone
- sex drive

The hypothalamus also controls the pituitary gland—the king of hormonal secretion. It is about the size of a small pea. These structures are vital for life in that they control most of our "vegetative" functions and drive states.

4. The Emotional Limbic System

Stimulate a section of a cat's hypothalamus and you'll see a sudden hissing and frenzied attack. Stimulate a different section and you'll find a purring kitty who'll want to sit on your lap. But both these behaviors have taken place in a vacuum. In neither case has the cat been provoked; it isn't angry—nor is it necessarily loving. Yes, the cat has most definitely "acted out" a behavioral response, but without any underlying emotion.

That's where the limbic system comes in. Found just below the higher functioning parts of the brain, this network of nerve cells literally provides us with the capacity to feel; it supplies the emotional tone of our actions. It adds the depth missing in the cat's "sham rage," in its empty purr. Thanks to the limbic system, we can feel true anger, sadness, joy, and elation. Because it's nestled right below the more cerebral, associative parts of the brain, the limbic system insures that emotions reach our conscious thoughts—and our thoughts affect our emotions. Both the limbic systems and the cerebral cortex are actively involved in influencing one another.

5. The Hippocampus and the Amygdala: Memories Are Made of This

They might sound like lands peopled by furry hobbits, magic, and wizards, but, in reality, the hippocampus and the amygdala are responsible for much of what we remember.

The hippocampus looks like a seahorse; it is located in the front of our brain. The hippocampus is directly connected to our senses, to touch, sight, sound, smell—and to our limbic system.

Thanks to its capacity to pick up, say, the vision of a bright summer day, its flowery scent wafting through a breeze, and its ability to connect this vision with a memory of a similar summer day in '72, one it's been storing for nearly twenty years, the hippocampus can "trigger" the limbic system into action, evoking the emotion of nostalgia.

And this emotion, in turn, helps "trigger" the cerebral, thinking areas of the brain where the hippocampus is located—which will open the floodgates on the past and all the thoughts, promises, and long ago dreams the past implies.

This rush of memory and its emotional images are helped along by the amygdala—which sits right in the middle of the limbic system itself.

But there is more to memory than emotion. Storing, cueing, retrieving, learning—all these aspects of memory, both short-term and long-term, can be found in. . . .

6. The Civilized Cerebral Cortex

Call it "gray power"—because it's the part of the brain that separates us from lower animals. It's here that we organize and abstract, communicate and appreciate, create and analyze, depending on which area of the cerebral cortex is involved.

But before we go on to these different sections, it's important to keep in mind that higher brain functions do their work in the *cortex*—which "merely" covers and clings to the brain. It's a blanket made of nerves, an eighth-of-an-inch-thick layer of billions and billions of cells. The cortex is completely uninspiring-looking, gray, and drab, but don't be fooled—this "blanket" of nerve cells holds what makes us human, what makes us individuals. Underneath it, warm and snug, is the chunky, white *cerebrum*. In order to increase its surface area the cortex wrinkles and rolls over the white matter—giving our brains their classic appearance.

Now that we've "covered" this distinction, let's go back to the sections of the cerebral cortex—which we call lobes. Think of this entire area of your brain with a line down the middle, dividing it in half. And, as if a magic marker had really been at work, you do indeed have two of the lobes I'll be describing below—one on the right side and one on the left. Each one has specific functions; each one can be injured—and result in different malfunctions. Let's go over these lobes now:

FRONTAL LOBES

These are known as the "seats" of the personality. The frontal lobes supervise many activities. True "CEOs" are responsible for all our executive functioning—from organizing to analyzing, from planning to decision-making, from staying focused to retrieving memory.

If a person's frontal lobes are damaged, it can hurt his or her ability to plan, to understand an idea or a new situation. He can become easily distracted. Her attention may be scattered.

THE OCCIPITAL (OR VISUAL) LOBES

Located in the back of the Cerebral Cortex, these lobes take information from our eyes and analyze what we are seeing. Damage here can result in cortical blindness.

THE TEMPORAL LOBES

You guessed it, these are located near our temples. You'll find the auditory cortex here, a small poker-chip lookalike that makes sense out of what we hear. They're also home for certain perceptions and memories. Damage to the temporal lobes can result in language, recent memory loss, and emotional problems.

BRAIN STORMING

The Animal Kingdom

Take away our prefrontal cortex and we virtually eliminate our human selves, our brains become the equal of an Arctic polar bear or the family cat. Peel the entire cortex away and our brains would be the same as those of snakes.

Dr. Paul MacLean, a brain researcher, claims that we have three separate brains that illuminate our relationship with our ancestors. The first "brain" is connected to the upper brainstem. Here are our neurons responsible for self-preservation—and our mating, hunting, and fighting instincts.

The second brain involves the limbic system—which reflects our bond to the mammal world. Here are our emotions, those feelings that guide our behavior. Injury to this area results in a regression back to the "first" brain, to more reptilian modes of action.

The third brain is the neo-cortex—which is all ours. The neo-cortex is the home for self-awareness, for problem-solving, for conceptualizing the future—all of which helps our other two "brains" in their ongoing battle to survive. It is also the place where insight is created, where we learn to understand, cope with, and help others and our selves.

This ability for self-awareness, coupled with our extraordinary language functioning, is what separates us from other mammals and the reptile world. It is what makes us uniquely human.

THE PARIETAL LOBES

They get their name from the Latin word for "forming the sides." You'll find these lobes between the frontal and occipital lobes and above the temporal lobe. But don't be deceived by their position. The parietal lobes serve an important function in bringing letters together as words—and turning words into thought. In fact, injuries to the parietal lobes can create amnesia, abnormalities in sensation, and neglect syndromes.

THE MAN WITH TWO BRAINS

We've all heard references like "She's really right-brained" for offbeat artists—or "He's really left-brained" for computer wizards. And it's true that the two hemispheres of the brain are different. Although they are mirror images of each other, they do possess different functions. But our right brains and left brains are not as opposite in as simple a way as was first thought. Basically each side works together, in sync—but each one uses a different strategy.

Here's an example: The left brain gives a person the ability to speak, but the right brain gives that speech its color, its drama, and inflection.

The *corpus callosum* is a network of nerves that connects these two hemispheres, enabling them to communicate with each other. When this "bridge" is severed, the right and left work independently, as if the other didn't exist. For example, one man whose corpus callosum was severed had been a talented artist. When he used his right hand to draw a horse (which, because each side of the brain controls the *opposite* side of the body, meant that his left brain was in charge), he depicted the exact replica of a horse, perfect in every detail—save one. It was a flat drawing; it had no spark. But when he used his left hand to draw the horse (which meant that his right-hemisphere was working), he created a complete abstraction. Yet, although this picture held no direct resemblance to a horse—no hoofs, no tail, no mane—it was immediately identifiable as "horse." It held the essence, the soul, missing in the left-brain drawing.

BRAIN STORMING

Moody Twos

Research conducted by Drs. Stewart Dimond and Linda Farrington found that the right hemisphere is involved more in negative emotions, the anxieties and fears we feel, while the left hemisphere is responsible more for our positive feelings—our laughter, joy, and sense of well-being. In fact, damage to our right brain can actually cause us to feel euphoric, as if we didn't have a care in the world.

It's important to know these different landmarks of the brain because damage to any area can help explain why someone is "not himself." But A doesn't always lead directly to B. Like most relationships in life, it all comes down to...

COMMUNICATION

Not all functions of the central nervous system are localizable to discrete brain sites. In fact, much of the disability that results from traumatic brain injury, or TBI, is related to a breakdown in communication between its parts—a disconnection, if you will, of "higher" controlling ones from lower "drive" producing ones.

Just as we dial a phone to talk to someone, so, too, does the brain have "telephone lines" that connect every part of itself to another part—and the entire central nervous system. These "party lines" are nerve cells called *neurons*. They carry messages through both electricity and chemical conductors. Here's how:

An electrical impulse, carrying, say, our message *hot-pain* will travel along a neuron—until it gets to the edge of the cell. There, in front of it, is a small space in the road called a *synapse*. Think of it as a river without a bridge. The electrical impulse cannot cross the "river." In order to get across the synapse to the next neuron and continue carrying its message, the impulse must change from an electrical "car" to a chemical "boat" or, in scientific terms, a *neurotransmitter*. Once the neurotransmitter "sails" across the synapse, it can convert back to electricity and continues to scurry through the new neuron to the next synapse—where this electrochemical process will again take place.

The neurotransmitters themselves are silent until stimulated, "quietly" waiting like docked boats in vesicles near the synapse. Only one specific electrical stimulus will activate a specific neurotransmitter. Similarly, only a specific neurotransmitting chemical will activate a specific synapse in the next cell. If this wasn't complicated enough, think of all this activity occurring simultaneously, fast and furious, with many different parts of the brain shouting orders and becoming involved. It's as if our brains are filled with millions of tiny locks and keys, continuously opening and closing when the fit is right.

Although the messages themselves can pertain to everything from hunger to hot, from worry to wonder, from deciding to take out a twenty at the cash machine to guilt about your mother, there is one basic brain communication theme:

NEUROTRANSMITTERS GENERALLY INHIBIT, NOT EXCITE

On the whole, the messages traveling through our brains are saying, "Calm down!" Higher cortical structures tend to modulate and inhibit lower ones. Although the lower and more central areas of the brain produce important drive states that keep our bodies functioning, a hallmark of our humanness is our ability to inhibit and control our impulses until such time as it is appropriate to gratify them.

Unfortunately, these inhibitory messages often originate in the frontal lobes of the cerebral cortex—which are very vulnerable to injury. This is why many brain-injured patients become aggressive, and why they suddenly seem to behave inappropriately. This characteristic of brain injury has so many ramifications for both patient and family alike that I'll be discussing it in depth later on. But, for now, remember that understanding is part of the rehabilitation process, and, by reading through this chapter, you have begun that first step.

*   *   *

In brief, then, this is how the brain functions. Unfortunately, physiology can only help us understand so much. Even as we pinpoint the various neurotransmitters and the electrical impulses sweeping throughout the brain, even as we stimulate and study our memories and emotions, our sleep patterns and our drive states, there is always a part of us that no one else sees, a part of us that is not behavior, that is not a steady heartbeat, a breath in and out, a thought, a cry. It is the self—and it is bigger than all of our chemicals and electrical configurations combined.

Our essence proves, beyond a shadow of a doubt, that the brain is much more than the sum of its parts; that we, our personalities, are more than statistics and facts.

Nowhere is this more apparent than when the brain is injured—and the self is transformed, a person is changed, sometimes forever.

Without further ado, let us see how.

TWO

WHEN BRAIN INJURY OCCURS

"Do you remember how you felt before your accident?"
"I was on top of the world."

—From an interview with a brain-injured patient at the Neurobehavioral Institute of Houston

Billy was determined to take care of the headlight on his antique car before he went to sleep that night. It was only seven o'clock, and the sun was barely set. He realized he needed some parts and, since it was Friday night, he knew the local hardware store would be open for at least another half hour. Rather than walk the half-mile, Billy decided to ride his bicycle. He checked his wallet, hopped on the seat and rode off. He didn't even tell his folks he was leaving; he expected to be back in fifteen minutes at the most.

There was Billy, sailing along on roads he'd ridden on since he was a toddler. But tonight was different. Tonight, fate provided one of its insidious tricks. Because it was dark, Billy didn't see the pothole looming up in front of him. His bike hit the depression at twenty-five miles an hour; Billy sailed over the handlebars and fell onto the side of the road. His unprotected head hit the curb.

Billy remembered "coming to." He was a bit dazed; he had some cuts and scrapes. Shaking his head, he dusted off his jeans, picked up his bike, and managed to ride home.

When he told his parents what had happened, his mother took his temperature. His father checked his arms and legs. Nothing was broken. He had no fever; he wasn't flushed, and except for the scrape on his forehead he looked all right. Billy showered and went to sleep; his antique car was forgotten for the night.

But, although he showed no outward signs of illness, Billy's problems were just beginning. The next morning, he couldn't get up. His mother had a hard time arousing him; he finally managed to get out of bed. Since it was Saturday, he spent much of the day hanging out around the house. No one gave it much thought throughout the weekend. Billy was a little tired, had an episode of vomiting or two, and headache, that's all.

However, Monday was a different story. In fact, he found the next few days in school difficult; he was confused and anxious. Billy felt a sense of vague foreboding that he couldn't place. Billy just couldn't think in class. He had headaches; he felt dizzy.

After a few days, Billy's personality went through a change. He became excited; he couldn't sleep. His appetite went down and he became hyperactive. His parents, apprehensive and concerned, took him to the family doctor—who told them that Billy had fractured his skull when he fell off his bike, but that it was healing nicely. There was nothing all that "physically" wrong with Billy.

Despite early hopes to the contrary, Billy's problems grew worse. He became angrier and angrier. Instead of the considerate boy they raised, his parents found themselves living with a "new" person in the house. The day Billy took a gun and shot a vase three feet from his mother was the final straw. His parents brought him to the Neurobehavioral Institute, where we discovered that Billy had not only fractured his skull in his accident. He had clearly injured his brain.

Billy was in the throes of a previously undiagnosed traumatic brain injury and he needed help....

Billy's tragedy is only one of the thousands that occur each year—each one as unique as the person involved. The fact is that traumatic brain injury isn't always the end result, nor do its symptoms have to show up immediately. Someone else might have flown over the handlebars, hit his head, and left the scene with a clean bill of health. On the other hand, someone else might have lost consciousness and gone into a deep coma.

But as varied as the end result and its symptoms are, there are some brain injury truths that are constant.

BRAIN STORMING

Bicycle Helmets Can Save Lives

It's true beyond a shadow of a doubt. Bicycle accidents cause 1300 deaths per year—mainly from head injuries. And half of these deaths are in children between the ages of 6 and 16. But these deaths could have been prevented if the victims had been wearing helmets. Here's proof:

- In a study of 235 people who were brain-injured while riding a bike, 7 percent were wearing headgear—but a whopping 93 percent were not.
- Of 99 cyclists with serious brain injury, only 4 percent wore helmets.
- Riders wearing helmets have 88 percent less chance of getting a brain injury.

In short: there's no excuse not to go out and buy helmets for your children when they begin to ride bikes. And pick one up for yourself while you're at it.

Skull and Bones

When you look at a typical skeleton's skull, one of its most notable features (besides the "scary" factor) is its smoothness. But that's the outside. Inside is a different story. The skull's interior surface, especially the area near your forehead and above your ears is bony; it's full of ridges and crevices. Most of the time, this doesn't bother your brain. It's happily bobbing about like Jell-O in a sea of cerebral spinal fluid.

But when you fall, crash through a windshield, or violently hit your head, your brain will literally get "shaken up," jiggling, banging, and rebounding against the hard ridges of its skull container.

Unfortunately, this means that your brain will more

than likely hit those bony ridges and crevices around your forehead and ears—exactly where your two "higher functioning" frontal and temporal lobes are located. Damage here, as we have already mentioned, can result in behavioral, cognitive, and emotional problems.

If bruising of the brain occurs, medical professionals call this condition *contusional* injury and, in varying degrees, it's often seen in TBI when acceleration/deceleration damage has been done.

In fact, when a person has an accident involving the brain, it's almost impossible *not* to involve the frontal and temporal lobes. Even if Billy had fallen over his back wheel instead of his handlebars, the back of his head hitting the ground, he still would have received a blow to his higher-functioning lobes. Why? Because his brain would be "pitched" forward in its sea of fluid, the fall meeting, first, the back of his head, then, as the force of the fall propels his brain forward, the front. Shaking violently, the brain will move from back to front, like a ball against a concrete wall of skull. This is called *coup-contrecoup injury,* a fairly common assault in which blows and counterblows make their bruising marks on the brain.

SPREADING THE NEWS

But the blows of outrageous fortune are not the only paths to TBI. *Diffuse axonal injury* is a widespread assault that's caused by the release of toxic neurochemicals and the stretching and tearing nerve fibers in the brain go through when a victim's head is violently shaken. It's a microscopic "shock wave," as the battered brain actually twists and shifts around, its matter being pulled and stretched like a rubber band. Since the greatest force in rotational injury is downward, diffuse axonal injury usually results in damage to the brainstem—which is part of the brain that's necessary for basic survival, for breathing, for staying alert.

This "shock wave" of injury can also come home to roost in the corpus callosum—which, as we have seen in Chapter One, integrates the two hemispheres of the brain. A severed corpus callosum results in a separation of function of the right and left hemispheres. Like the artist with the divided brain hemispheres who tried to draw a horse, the two cannot come together.

Denial is often a symptom that crops up in right brain injury. One 39-year-old woman, paralyzed on her left side because of right hemisphere damage, saw her own "useless" left arm resting on her pillow and claimed it was her daughter's arm—not hers. Another patient, a man, ignored all the food on the left side of his plate. He simply didn't "see" it.

BRAIN STORMING

TBI Statistics

- Males are three times more likely than females to receive a brain injury
- 70 percent of all brain injuries happen in young adults under 30—with teens between 15 and 24 years old at the most risk.
- Head injuries are three times more likely in the unemployed.
- As a whole, people in the lower socioeconomic classes have more head injuries.
- A person who suffers from one brain injury is at a greater risk of suffering from another one.
- Alcoholics, drug abusers, and people suffering from psychiatric illnesses are at increased risk of brain injury.

AN OPEN AND SHUT CASE

In addition to these three primary brain injuries, physicians also refer to traumatic brain injury with the words *open* or *closed*. These terms are used to describe the general categories of TBI:

- An *open* injury to the brain is caused by, say, a bullet that has entered the brain through the skull. It is an injury that has penetrated the brain from outside.
- A *closed* head injury occurs when the brain has not been penetrated. The trauma is all internal, from the bouncing and pounding of the brain against the interior side of the skull.

But whether an open or closed injury, contusional, or even a diffuse axonal injury, brain injury can result in a myriad of secondary problems, including brain swelling, a lack of oxygen, and bleeding. All these continue to cause damage to the brain and can lead to cognitive and emotional problems. I will discuss these different conditions and symptoms at length in Chapter Three and throughout Part II of this book.

PROBLEMS IN THE MAKING

The physical results of TBI can be uncomfortable and even catastrophic until they are accepted. But the headaches, the lack of coordination, the dizziness, the inability to walk, for perhaps a few weeks or months—none of these will hold most people back forever. It's the behavioral problems that do people in.

Language. Logic. Speech. Emotions. Understanding. Memory. These are some of the bitter secondary problems that can crop up. Like Billy, they can become a reality a few days after an injury. They can sometimes be discovered immediately. And sometimes the affected parts of the brain are so microscopic in size that the injuries don't show up on any diagnostic test—even though they can cause such damage.

Here's a telling example of memory loss excerpted from Oliver Sacks's *The Man Who Mistook His Wife for a Hat:*

Dr. Sacks had been interviewing a 49-year-old man who had amnesia. He not only was unable to remember things that just happened in the present, but he was actually reliving the past in his mind. The dialogue went like this:

"What year is this, Mr. G.?," I asked, concealing my perplexity under a casual manner.

"Forty-five, man. What do you mean?" He went on. "We've won the war, FDR's dead, Truman's at the helm. There are great times ahead."

"And you, Jimmie, how old would you be?"

Oddly, uncertainly he hesitated a moment, as if engaged in calculation.

"Why, I guess I'm nineteen, Doc. I'll be twenty next birthday."

Dr. Sacks showed Mr. G. a mirror which he knew would have been *"the height of cruelty had there been any possibility of Jimmie's remembering."*

But Jimmie didn't. Although he panicked at the sight of his aging face in the mirror, Jimmie not only didn't remember what he had seen in the mirror, but he didn't remember Dr. Sacks when he returned to the room two minutes later.

As this example so profoundly shows, traumatic brain injury affects people where they live: their minds.

Think about it. If you become blind, but your brain is okay, your brain will help you adapt to not seeing. You think, Something's happened. I'm blind. What am I going to do? How am I going to cope?

But with brain injury, the one organ that would help you cope is the one that's hurt. Like Jimmie G. in the Oliver Sacks example, its survivors themselves don't—and often can't—recognize the depths of their difficulties.

This is both a blessing and a curse. It's a blessing because, unlike the blind person, a TBI victim is not immediately devastated by his loss. But it is a curse because when he wants to re-enter the community or get a job or simply become a member of his family again, he's going to have trouble. He doesn't think anything's wrong with him—but everyone around him does. He keeps repeating the same mistakes. He becomes frustrated by not being able to do simple things, like initiate new activities or plan for the next day. Chances are, there'll be family conflict because of his unawareness—and he may not understand what they mean when they say, "You're different."

Often, the TBI victim becomes more and more discouraged. Damaged brain cells, and external stress—all take their toll, working psychologically and physically to spiral him down, down into a depression. In his pain, he might turn to alcohol or drugs, abusing himself. . . .

It's a vicious cycle, one that feeds upon itself. There can be many sources, but the symptoms all have a common link: confusion, pain, and disability.

But it doesn't have to be this way. Understanding is important—and there is more to be learned before we go on to rehabilitation and recovery. First, let's examine the different types of brain injuries. . . .

THREE

TYPES OF BRAIN INJURY

"I have to try harder now."

—Rob, age 47, a TBI patient at the
Neurobehavioral Institute of Houston

- Whenever Rosemary tries to speak, few words come out, and those that do are garbled. Her hand gestures, her tone of voice—all imply that she knows what she's trying to communicate, but no one can understand her.
- As an accountant, Bruce used to spend each day poring over figures and spreadsheets. Although he can still do simple problems with a calculator, more complex math leaves him muddled and confused.
- Susan is 58 years old, but she cannot tell you the correct time. She has difficulty walking and cannot find her way to her room; at times she is incontinent.
- Gary was once an enthusiastic, energetic teen. But he just spent his eighteenth birthday staring off into space; he looks frozen in time.

There is one common element in these tragic tales: each person, young or old, is brain-injured. But, although their symptoms might appear similar, each person's brain has been injured in a different way—and each require a somewhat different treatment approach:

Rosemary had a stroke in her sixties that involved a

part of the left hemisphere of her brain; her treatment plan concentrates on teaching her to translate her needs to others by using a "communication board."

Bruce had been in a car accident; he suffered a closed head injury which affected his frontal lobes. He needs intensive neuropsychological and vocational rehabilitation.

Susan has dementia, and, after a careful evaluation, it was discovered that she has severe deficiency of vitamin B-12. Once the cause of the problem was identified, therapy was begun with an injectible form of this vitamin.

Gary has another type of frontal brain injury which produces depression, apathy, and decreased drive. A search is begun to find anything that will motivate him. His family shares his former interests with the treatment team, and systematically his increasing responsiveness is "rewarded" with these reinforcers.

In short, brain injury can be either the result of disease or a sudden accident. This book is essentially about traumatic brain injury, but, since symptoms and treatments can overlap, I will very briefly discuss the diseases of the brain that can cause disability, starting with . . .

Parkinson's Disease

This illness is named after London physician James Parkinson who first described and studied the disease in 1817. It is a movement disorder, one that involves speech and walking difficulties, shaking and tremors—a condition whereby push and pull are constantly at odds, eventually freezing a person into a mute immobility. Today, scientists have discovered that this disease is caused by a deficiency of the neurotransmitter dopamine in the brain. Without enough dopamine, some neurons can't come to life; they remain inactive while others overpower them. In his inspiring book *Awakenings* (and as depicted in the movie of the same name), Oliver Sacks administers a synthesized dopamine precursor, L-Dopa, to patients who suffered from a type of Parkinson's disease that had left them frozen. The results were startling. Men and women who had been "asleep" for nearly twenty years became rejuvenated. Like Rip Van Winkle, they literally "woke" up to a brand new world.

Senility and Alzheimer's Disease

As Joanne Woodward so dramatically portrayed in the television movie *Do You Remember Love?*, Alzheimer's disease is devastating to both the victim and his or her loved ones. Both this and "senility" are aptly labeled dementia. Approximately 5 percent of all persons over sixty-five suffer from this disease, which at first affects the individual's recent memory. People may forget what they had for breakfast and lose track of appointments while easily recalling the events of their wedding day thirty years before. Eventually, the name for "teapot," the direction of the bedroom, the route one takes to work each day—all these facts become cloudy. Finally, as the deterioration continues and all cognitive and behavioral processes become affected, people seem to lose their "senses."

Studies have found that abnormal proteins and neurons in both the cerebral cortex and the hippocampus presumably cause this form of dementia. A malfunctioning neurotransmitter called acetylcholine has also been discovered to be a contributing culprit. Various medications are being tested that will increase production of acetycholine in the brain and, therefore, hopefully improve the individual's memory.

Strokes

This is a simple word with a deadly impact. Cerebral vascular accident (CVA), or its more common name of stroke, occurs when one or more blood vessels in the brain gets blocked or bursts open. Depending on its severity and location of the blood vessels affected, stroke victims will usually suffer from one or more disabilities, including paralysis or weakness on one side of the body, mood swings, swallowing difficulties, language problems, agitation, and impulsiveness. About 600,000 Americans every year are maimed by strokes and need the physical, speech, and neuropsychological therapies that rehabilitation centers offer.

Tumors

Tumors are growths of abnormal, rapidly dividing cells that interfere with normal body function. They can appear anywhere in the body, including the brain, and can be benign or malignant. Depending on its location and its cell type, a tumor can alter any bodily function, from balance to perception, from memory to mood, from coordination to language comprehension. Death is not always the ultimate result of a brain tumor. Today's advances in diagnostic testing, in laser surgery, and chemotherapy can all help reduce the morbidity associated with this disease.

Cardiac Arrest

A person may survive a heart attack, but his brain could still be injured in the race against the clock. During cardiac arrest, the brain's oxygen supply is cut off; this is called anoxia. Unless the person having the attack is quickly revived, brain cells begin to die, especially in the very active parts of the CNS that require the most oxygen—resulting in memory loss, poor judgment, faulty thinking, and regressed behavior.

But even under these dire circumstances, there is new hope. Studies have shown that brain cells live longer than previously thought. Instead of minutes, many neurons live for hours after their oxygen supply is cut off, and research done by Dr. Dennis W. Choi of Stanford University is showing that neurons can be "plugged" with an injected drug that both "locks" in their oxygen-supplying glucose and keeps the toxic environment that causes brain cell death at bay—at least for the time it takes to fully resuscitate the individual and have his heart beat regularly again.

All of these injuries occur in fully developed adults. They can happen suddenly, without warning, or they can slowly and subtly show the signs of problem behavior early on. But each one also has its own set of symptoms, its own natural history, and its own set of handicapping conditions that require differing treatment strategies.

Traumatic brain injury is different. Yes, it occurs suddenly. It interrupts a normal life. It leaves a person significantly different—just as any other brain injury does. But TBI goes one step further: a person can have *all* the symptoms I've just described for each individual illness—and he can have them all at the same time. He can be physically incapacitated. He can have trouble thinking. His mood swings can come alarmingly fast and furious. He can lose control. In short, a person with traumatic brain injury needs rehabilitation for every facet of his being, in every arena that makes him a whole person, and because TBI is the result of a terrible outside force, an external twist of fate, it has its own brand of surprise, disability, and pain. But, as with all of life's viscissitudes, there are different degrees of severity. In fact, there are four. Let's go over these now.

DEGREE OF PAIN #1: MILD BRAIN INJURY

The most common of all brain injuries, it's usually the result of falls, car accidents, and tackles on the football field. If someone you know has suffered from mild brain injury, he will be unconscious briefly, if at all and generally he will have "come to" by the time you've reached the hospital emergency entrance. However, he may remain confused or have difficulty remembering things for up to an hour. He'll most likely complain of headache, nausea, and dizziness—the result often of brain swelling and the release of excessive excitatory neurotransmitters. As a rule, these early symptoms clear up within a few weeks or months.

BRAIN STORMING

Preventing Sports Injuries

All good coaches should have their players:
- Use protective gear—always
- Train under supervision
- Avoid dangerous horseplay—and dangerous maneuvers on the playing field
- Undergo regular physical examinations
- Participate in and attend periodic counseling sessions that emphasize "fair play"
- Rehearse emergency procedures to be used when a teammate is injured

---

Unfortunately, there are always exceptions to every rule—and that includes my description of mild brain injury. The fact is that the term "mild" may be a misnomer; this type of injury is not always as innocent and clear-cut

BRAIN STORMING

Figures of Speech

The word *concussion* is tossed around a great deal when traumatic brain injury is diagnosed. In actuality, a concussion is nothing more than another way of saying the brain has been violently shaken or jarred such that there is an alteration in the person's level of awareness.

Another word often heard associated with TBI is *coma*. Besides its use as a title for the bestselling book by Robin Cook, coma means a deep unconsciousness. In fact, it is literally taken from the Greek word for "deep sleep." The length and type of coma can reflect the damage done by a concussion. Eye opening, motor responses, and verbal responses are all used to determine how "deep" a coma is. (See Chapter Ten for more on comas.)

as it first appears. Although research in diagnostic testing has made incredible advances, there can be "microscopic" brain injury that isn't picked up by the newest technologies, or slight neurological malfunctioning that, undetected, can produce memory problems, irritability, depression, restlessness, and a lack of focus several weeks to several months down the road—the late symptoms of mild brain injury.

These unpleasant symptoms can begin an insidious chain of events: conflicts at home, reprimands on the job, rejection from friends. These painful traumatic events, in turn, create secondary psychological problems—on top of the still undiscovered neurological ones. Severe depression, anxiety, irritability, alcohol and substance abuse—all these behavioral disorders, although born in that "mild" brain injury, now have a life of their own that must be treated.

More grim news: This condition, called post-concussive syndrome, or more properly, concussion syndrome, is not usually recognized until a person has lost a job or failed in school, until a spouse has "walked out" in exasperation, until the victim himself has become so psychologically impaired that he, too, believes himself a "failure" in life. Confused and depressed, he doesn't understand what is going on—or why he can't perform the way he did.

Here's a real-life example of the tragic aftermath of mild brain injury, as discussed in the Washington Business Group on Health's *Business and Health* magazine:

A.T. was a 34-year-old advertising vice-president; she earned more than $100,000 a year. But one night, on her way home from work, her car collided with a truck. A.T. was only unconscious for twenty minutes, but because she was a bit dazed and confused, she was admitted to the hospital to undergo a few days of tests. Nothing was found and she was told to go home and rest for a few days.

But nothing would hold A.T. down. She was back on the job two weeks later—although something wasn't quite right. She didn't feel like the same person; something was bothering her, something she couldn't place. Professional to the core, A.T. tried to downplay her problems. When she was tired or confused, she pushed it away. When she forgot routine business meetings, she ignored it. But when she was challenged or asked why she had made a certain business decision, A.T. couldn't control herself. She would get angry or upset—and push her colleagues even further away than they already were. Finally, four months later, her boss fired her; he hadn't realized that the changes in A.T. were directly related to the "minor" accident she had had months before.

Unfortunately, neither did A.T. Unemployed, confused, depressed, and drinking heavily, A.T. became obsessed with getting her job back. Additional neurological tests showed that she was still extremely bright, articulate, and capable, but this time around, they did show that she had some very subtle cognitive impairments, difficulties that would hinder her "executive" capabilities.

But A.T. refused to accept this diagnosis. She wanted to be a vice-president again—or nothing. She was admitted to a hospital where she is currently learning to accept, understand—and even like—her new self.

DEGREE #2: MODERATE BRAIN INJURY

When this diagnosis is given, it's because a person has been unconscious or experienced post-traumatic amnesia for up to 24 hours. More than likely, a moderately brain-injured person will be transferred to a rehabilitation program once the medical crisis caused by the accident has passed. Although resulting cognitive, emotional, and behavioral problems vary from person to person, most moderately brain-injured people are not ready to go back to work for at least six months. In fact, one study found that up to two-thirds of moderately brain-injured persons were unable to return to work a year after their accidents.

Some of its symptoms include tremors, lack of coordination, weakness, language difficulties, and problems with memory, perception, planning, and judgment.

DEGREE #3: SEVERE BRAIN INJURY

A person suffers from severe brain injury when he or she has been in a coma (deep unconsciousness) for more than one day. Rehabilitation is generally required, and often needs to continue on an outpatient basis as well. In addition to cognitive, emotional, and behavioral training, severely brain-injured persons must be retaught how to be independent on the most basic levels. Living skills, social skills, and independent, personal grooming—these are the goals of the severely brain-injured.

If a severely brain-injured person is able to go back to work, it may be in a reduced capacity—and perhaps only after several years of rehabilitation.

DEGREE #4: CATASTROPHIC BRAIN INJURY

This type of brain injury is exactly what it sounds like: catastrophic. A person brought down by this severe a brain injury might wake, sleep and breathe—but it will only be a "twilight" kind of awareness. Catastrophically brain-injured people will be in a coma for weeks or months; they cannot speak, follow commands, or even understand what is being said to them. Unfortunately, rehabilitation may become a lifelong process.

Although I've tried to explain these four levels of brain injury in as simple terms as possible, none of them are as clear-cut as they might seem. There is no black-and-white scenario—or an absolutely certain outcome. Some people have made startling recoveries from severe traumatic brain injury—even after they'd been given a poor prognosis. Inroads have been made with people that, for months appeared to be severely impaired. Even after a person's brain has been soothed, healed, and retrained, a positive environment can continue to work wonders, increasing awareness and ability in all areas.

In short, hope is ever-present. Not foolish hope, not wishful thinking, but a realistic belief that with proper care and rehabilitation, progress can be made.

And, in the name of progress, it's time now to dispel old tales, separate fact from fancy, and put some brain injury myths to rest once and for all.

FOUR

BRAIN INJURY MYTHS

"Within the book and volume of my brain."

—William Shakespeare, *Hamlet,* Act I, Scene 5

Ignorance is not bliss—especially when it comes to traumatic brain injury. It's simple: The more you know, the more you can understand. The more you understand, the more you can accept. And, the more you can accept, the more progress can be made in rehabilitation.

In the name of that progress, here are the realities behind the most common brain injury myths, the hindering beliefs that, in my years of academic practice and as medical director of the Neurobehavioral Institute of Houston, have cropped up again and again:

MYTH #1: "Brain Injury Can Be Recognized and Detected Immediately"

Roger is a patient of mine at our Houston program. In 1978, he'd been driving a company truck; he hit a guard rail and broke his arm and leg. He also suffered from a minor closed head injury, but it took two years for it to be diagnosed. Within those years, Roger lost his job. He couldn't sustain any relationships. "Girls got scared of me," he told me during his admission interview. "I had this temper, you know. But it was like I couldn't control it and I didn't know why."

Like Billy, the tragic bicycle rider, or A.T., the executive who lost her job and took to drink, minor head injury isn't always discovered at the time of the accident. Unlike a fractured bone or a bleeding wound, head injuries can be "invisible." The amount of damage can't always be seen— even with our advanced diagnostic tools. Nor can we immediately pinpoint exactly which areas of the brain are affected. Damage in the frontal lobe area can have far-reaching tentacles, causing neurological and chemical imbalances in the limbic system, the temporal, and the parietal lobes. On the other hand, the damage can be self-contained, causing only slight, temporary injury to the frontal systems.

In short, brain injury can have a life of its own. When someone you love is injured in an accident, it's crucial to pay attention to his moods, his conversations, and his habits for several months down the road. Communicate. If anything, however slight, seems different or wrong, contact your doctor. Early detection can make all the difference between a downward spiral and health.

MYTH #2: "The Healing Process Only Takes a Few Months"

Wrong. More than anything else, brain injury takes time to heal. It can't be rushed. Swelling must subside. Bruises must heal. Disrupted neurons must be soothed and repaired. Neurotransmitters must be given a chance to re-equilabrate.

All these processes take time. It is not uncommon for even those with minor brain injury to require long-term neurobehavioral rehabilitation. More severe damage can mean extended hospital and outpatient treatment for a year, or even longer. Be patient. Like broken legs and broken hearts, healing cannot be rushed.

MYTH #3: "His Brain Injury Is Just an Excuse to Do Whatever He Wants to Do. It's All in His Head"

What came first, the chicken or the egg? A study of 145

people suffering from minor brain injury found that 38.9 percent continued to have symptoms of memory loss, fatigue, depression, and sensitivity to alcohol one year after their accident. Women had more of these symptoms than men. So did those who viewed themselves as "victims," blaming their employers or large organizations for their accidents. But the study also found a correlation between these "psychological symptoms" and the amount of neurological damage at the time of the accident.

As this research shows, the answer has nothing to do with what came first—or last. Both psychology and physiology work in concert, one affecting the other, necessitating "holistic" treatment that addresses both physical and mental problems simultaneously.

BRAIN STORMING

In 1848, 25-year-old Phineas Gage was on the job, supervising a Rutland and Burlington Railroad work crew. They were blasting rock from a gorge. Mr. Gage had dropped a tamping iron into a hole filled with gunpowder. The powder went off, and the iron hit Gage right between the eyes. It went through his frontal lobes and back out the other side. However, despite the severity of his accident Phineas Gage did not die. In fact, he actually walked up the stairs to his hotel room in town. But he was no longer himself. He became a "lost soul," the balance between his thoughts and his emotions destroyed. He'd go into complete rages; he became stubborn, a petulant child. His intellectual, executive abilities to manage others, to create enthusiasm and solve problems, was gone.

Phineas Gage became a drifter. Twelve years, six months, and eight days after the tamping iron seared through his brain, he died.

MYTH #4: "Even After Major Injury, a Person Can Completely Recover"

Here is a fact that must be addressed: there is no such thing as full recovery following a significant brain injury.

Yes, a person improves—but subtle changes often persist even in the best of scenarios. And studies have found that in many ways improvement is dependent on the severity of the initial injury. Mildly brain-injured persons can show vast improvement in a few months to a year—or, as we have seen, they can suffer from "concussive syndrome" for years after their accident. Moderate and severely injured people will improve more slowly.

But improvement does not imply complete recovery. The reality is that brain injury, more times than not, involves some permanent disabilities. They may be slight, but they are there. It's crucial for you to not only be aware of what can be a chronic condition, but accept it as well, creating new goals, new life, from the "ashes."

MYTH #5: "A Traumatic Brain Injury Almost Guarantees Malingering"

It's been my experience that brain-injured patients want to get better. They feel extremely frustrated; they want to go on with their lives. They rarely use their injury as an excuse to "hide" from the world.

But they can learn to be dependent. As with many other disabled people, they become used to others taking care of them. That's why independence training is stressed. Personal hygiene, laundry detail, washing dishes—all these help create an atmosphere of independent living and with it, an important sense of self-worth.

MYTH #6: "Except for Some Slight Disorientation, People Wake Up from Comas Raring to Go"

Picture this scene: The rain is hitting the hospital window. The brain-injured patient, lying in his bed for two months in a deep coma, suddenly sits up and looks at the woman sitting in the straight-backed chair by the bed. "Why did you try to kill me, Mary!" the patient shouts. The music swells and the episode of "My Favorite Soap Opera" cuts for a commercial. . . .

If only people could come out of comas like this, injury-free and ready to take on the world! Unfortunately, comas just don't work that way. The reality is that you're out of it for quite a while after waking up. You're spacey and maybe delirious. Maybe you're kicking and pulling at your intravenous lines. Or maybe you're lethargic and staring into space. In fact, you're often not even going to know who or where you are for weeks.

MYTH #7: "A Miracle Will Happen and She'll Be the Way She Was Before the Accident"

Researchers call it the Lourdes Phenomenon, the situation in which families, having difficulty facing their loved one's disability, hope for a miracle to occur. In pursuit of that dream, they will go from doctor to doctor, program to program, spending money, time and energy on something as elusive as eternal life.

It's true that some elements do make for improvement: a good therapist, a good rehabilitation program, a positive environmental "trigger" such as the start of a new relationship or a decent job. But, as we have seen, improvement does not mean full recovery. The clock cannot be turned back. Permanent limitations will not go away. The person you knew and loved is changed—and she's not going to come fully back. Instead of searching for a "cure," families must learn to change, too. They must learn to accept what is.

Myths are one thing—and reality is another. Let us now go on to the specific realities of brain injury, the sometimes "invisible" injurious assaults that can irrevocably change a person's life.

PART II

INJURIOUS ASSAULTS

FIVE

DETECTIVE WORK: DISCOVERING TBI

"We can do more. And we will, soon."

—Dr. Bruce H. Dobkin, neurologist

Here's an excerpt from a 1920s newspaper article, reprinted in *Awakenings* by Oliver Sacks:

> ASLEEP FOR THREE YEARS...
> *In The World and Yet Out*
> *From Our Own Correspondent*
> The tragic case of a man being in the world and yet out of it was described to me yesterday.
> This man, workless and homeless, more than three years ago walked into the West Highland Rest Home. He complained of being terribly tired, and it was obvious that his complaint was genuine. He simply could not keep awake.
> When the doctor examined him he found the man was suffering from sleeping sickness, and he was put to bed right away. He is still sleeping.

It's hard to believe, but during the 1920s there was a medical scare as terrifying as polio was in the 1950s, as AIDS is today. People called it the "sleeping sickness," but physicians knew it as encephalitis lethargica, a type of Parkinson's disease that turned well-balanced children and adults into violent, insolent, and aggressive "monsters" —almost overnight. Ultimately, these victims were left physically helpless, their movements frozen in a push-pull tension that, like two magnets, could never come together. They appeared asleep, frozen in time. As the movie *Awakenings* so poignantly depicted, the drug L-Dopa literally gave those suffering from encephalitis lethargica their lives back—after twenty or thirty years of "sleeping" in one institution or another.

But encephalitis lethargica is more than a fascinating glimpse through time. Not only did it make inroads into Parkinson's disease research, encephalitis lethargica also clearly demonstrated that diseases of the brain could produce disorders in behavior.

THE SLEEPING CONNECTION

After World War II, the worlds of neurology and psychiatry had moved far apart—despite the fact that Freud began his professional life as a neurologist. One had little to do with the other. Period. But people suffering from conditions such as encephalitis lethargica were found to have both neurological abnormalities *and* psychological ones. Inflamed lesions on the spinal cord and upper midbrain, an inordinately long sleep cycle, tremors—all these signaled neurological damage. But the child who became hyperactive in the later stages of the disease; the man who exhibited obsessive-compulsive behavior and movements, washing and rewashing his hands; the teen who became depressed—these were disorders of the mind. Without a doubt, encephalitis lethargica proved there was a connection between neurology and psychology.

Unfortunately, professionals in these two disciplines did not immediately join hands. Psychiatrists continued to believe that the psyche was a separate entity, working independently to create an individual's personality. Behaviorists took the view that action itself held the answers—and refused to delve deeper. Neurologists emphatically agreed that disorders of the mind were all a case of chemicals and cellular structure that went awry.

But, thanks to progress and advanced technologies, the lessons learned from encephalitis lethargica have been reassessed. We now know that mind and brain cannot be separated. Damage in the central nervous system will often lead to psychic damage.

The discipline of neuropsychiatry was reborn, with its more balanced belief that psychological processes are driven by a brain base.

But this balanced view would not have evolved if our knowledge of the brain had remained in...

ANCIENT TIMES

Galen was a Greek physician, practicing in the second century A.D. As court-appointed doctor to the gladiators, he learned firsthand how a lance's blow to the head could cause brain injury. Unfortunately, Aristotle was the reigning philosopher of the day, and he believed that the source of all thoughts and feelings was the heart. The brain was merely the receptacle for "animal spirit," conceived by the cosmos and carried throughout the body via a network of hollow nerve fibers. Even William Harvey, the scientist who discovered blood circulation, was reported to have said in 1616, "The brain is deemed the prince of all parts. However, there is no disputing the heart because its sway is wider, for the heart is seen in those creatures that want a brain."

Like a flat earth, this belief would last through the centuries. It would take a frog and a squid to change the way we felt about the brain.

ANIMAL TALES

He must have been much in demand as a dinner party guest, for Luigi Galvani would, after dessert was served, take out a frog and perform an experiment with electricity—and if a thunderstorm was imminent, so much the better! He'd attach a dissected frog to a table; a wire would go from its head to a metal rod on the balcony. He'd place another wire from the frog's foot to a well of water. As soon as the lightning flashed, lo and behold, the dead frog's muscle twitched, showing that "animal electricity" surged through the nerves in our brain.

From after-dinner exhibitions to the science lab, it soon became apparent that the brain generated a weak electrical current. But it was not until the 1930s that the specifics of electrochemical conversion would be discovered—thanks to a squid. The tubular appendage that allowed a squid to swim was one big nerve cell. When scientists inserted electrodes into this cell, they discovered that, at rest, there were separate charges surging through it—both positive and negative. Further squid experiments showed that all communication was the result of altering the charge in this "at rest" state.

BRAIN STORMING

Sakharov's Brain

Andrei Sakharov was the father of the Soviet hydrogen bomb and a human rights activist, a hero to some, a villain to others. But now he is dead at 68, and Russia is about to make amends—at least with his brain. His brain now currently resides at the Soviet Union's Brain Institute. But as Russian literature expert and publisher Ellendea Proffer told *USA Today,* "They have a long history of doing this, back to the last century. They're trying to find out what makes certain people brilliant. But this is special treatment reserved for extraordinary people."

Incidentally, back home, Albert Einstein's brain cells were recently used to study the aging process.

When this electric connection was combined with the dedicated work of scientists such as Carmillio Golgi, who in 1906 discovered that nerve cells were separated from each other by a synapse, the electrochemical neurotransmitting theory being tossed about in scientific circles became reality. And with this groundbreaking news came more clues and more detective work—leading to progress into the whys and wherefores of brain injury. Here are some examples:

- We now know that some neurotransmitters send inhibitory messages from one part of the brain to another, which can get disrupted when the brain is damaged. Under these circumstances neuronal communication becomes confused or impossible. Instead of the usual homeostatic control, our drives are likely to be expressed at inopportune times or in exaggerated form.

- To treat epilepsy, neurosurgeons in the 1940s would sever the corpus callosum "bridge" between the right and left hemispheres of the brain, thus preventing a seizure from moving from the left side to the right, and vice versa. Although the operation was successful and the seizures stopped, so did many of the integrated functions of the brain, which provided an opportunity to study the differing functions of the two hemispheres.

- A man who'd injured his head in a car accident seemed to have no brain damage, except for one thing: he no longer had any interest in sex. After careful diagnostic testing, his physician came to the conclusion that the man's injury damaged his hypothalamus—the small "pea" that gives the pituitary gland permission to secrete the sexual hormone GnRH. With the use of a special pump filled with GnRH, this man's hormone level was happily stabilized, but the story doesn't end here. This example demonstrates the fact that brain injury doesn't necessarily affect movement, intellectual functions, or moods. It can also affect our rhythms and our drives, sometimes in conjunction with other injury—and sometimes alone.

- A woman was so obsessive-compulsive that she could barely function. She spent most of her time in seemingly meaningless rituals, compulsions like washing her hands, walking back and forth to the door, counting to ten over and over again. She couldn't stop herself: all she could think about was death. She shot herself in the head and, lo and behold, she was no longer obsessive-compulsive. She had, in effect, given herself a "lobotomy." But the woman's visual perception was gone, as was her essence—again, terrible proof that some neuropsychiatric disorders do, in fact, have an organic basis.

- As we have seen, brain injury can give birth to depression, aggression, emotional pain, and substance abuse. In fact, one study found that 70 percent of all brain-injured people suffer from irritability and aggressiveness. Other studies have found that depression is quite common after brain injury. For not only is the person suddenly and overwhelmingly confronted with the physical, mental, and even social consequences of his injury, but those structures in the frontal area of the brain that control mood are often damaged as well. The good news is that the depression is usually more treatable now then ever before.

BRAIN STORMING

The Glasgow Coma Scale

Eye Opening

Spontaneously	4
To speech	3
To pain	2
None	1

Best Verbal Response

Oriented	5
Confused	4
Inappropriate words	3
Incomprehensible	2
None	1

Best Motor Response

Obey commands	6
Flexion (bending) withdrawal	5
Localize pain	4
Flexion to pain	3
Extension to pain	2
None	1

Total Score: 3 = profound coma
                 15 = mild brain injury

TESTING, TESTING

Studies have found that early intervention is crucial, not only for life-saving neurosurgery, but for successful rehabilitation. Therapy that begins in the hospital ward, even if a patient is still in a coma, may make all the difference in his ability to physically improve from brain injury.

This therapy begins with a thorough diagnosis. Although microscopic damage can stay hidden from view, today's technology has considerably narrowed the percentage of cases that slip through. Here, very briefly, are some of the diagnostic tests used in the evaluation of traumatic brain injury:

1. CAT Scan

Although this examination sounds more like a veterinarian's test, it looks, in actuality, like something from a sci-fi flick. A patient lies down inside a large white circular capsule as technicians take three-dimensional X-rays of her brain. By moving the cameras various "slices" of the brain can be viewed to help locate the anatomic pathology that results from an insult to the brain. Incidentally, CAT stands for computerized axial tomography. It is most commonly used in the emergency department to detect bleeding in the brain.

2. MRI

Magnetic resonance imaging is one of the newest brain-imaging diagnostic tools. Like CAT scans, MRI can pinpoint problem areas in the brain, but with more precision. Utilizing radio frequency pulses and the brain's hydrogen protons, MRI is able to convert the resulting electrical signals into a computerized picture of the brain, exposing minute detail that, prior to this test, would have gone undetected, especially in deep brain structures.

3. SPECT and PET Scans

These provide more than just anatomic information about the brain. In fact, both tests, although still research tools, tell the clinician about the functional capacity of the major brain areas. These techniques highlight abnormalities that may not show up on either CAT or MRI scans.

4. EEG

EEG is the short way of describing an electroencephalogram test. Here, electrodes attached to the scalp measure electrical impulses surging through the brain. Abnormal peaks and valleys or spikes on a printout would, for example, signify seizures.

5. Neuropsychological Testing

This is also a "functional" evaluation and is principally designed to test each area of the brain to see if it is performing as it should. Tests of attention, intellectual functioning, language and memory are often included in the battery administered to brain injury survivors. This is a lengthy evaluation usually requiring two days to administer and to score by psychologists specially trained in these techniques.

These are only a few of the diagnostic tools in use today. The more we learn about the brain, the more sophisticated our diagnostic capabilities. Every day, new tools are being created and tested, all of which help us define exactly where a brain injury has occurred and what functions it has impaired. (You'll read about more of these tests in later chapters.)

But our detective work is not yet done. A general overview of traumatic brain injury is one thing, but it's time to get more specific, to observe, close up, the symptoms that can crop up in TBI.

SIX

TBI: The Physical Factor

"I never thought it would happen to me."

—A paraplegic TBI patient at the
Neurobehavioral Institute of Houston

This is the way it happened: Joan had been settling into her new apartment in Boston's Back Bay. She was about to begin her residency at the prestigious Massachusetts General Hospital; her fiancé and she had just made wedding plans; money from a grant she'd been awarded was in the mail. Everything was going her way; it was a dream come true. In fact, Joan was so excited, so hyper, that if she didn't blow off some steam, she'd jump out of her skin. She decided to go out for a quick jog.

It worked. Four miles along the Charles in the settling dusk was enough to calm her down. Joan walked back to the townhouse where she lived. But as she entered her apartment, she heard a noise. She had interrupted a robbery in progress—in her own living room. It all happened so quickly that Joan couldn't identify the assailants. She was struck on the head from behind. She heard a voice say, "Let's get outta here." Then silence. She blacked out.

A neighbor coming up the stairs a few minutes later saw Joan's wide-open door. She peeked in and saw Joan, unconscious on the floor. She dropped her groceries, picked up the phone, and dialed the police.

Within fifteen minutes, Joan was in the emergency

room of the very hospital in which she was to begin her residency. She was beginning to come around, although her head was pounding and she felt disoriented. She was quickly examined. A CAT Scan and a neurological examination were performed. The diagnosis? A mild closed brain injury. She had suffered a concussion. Her brain was bruised both in its posterior and frontal areas from the "coup-contrecoup" action produced by the assault. (See Chapter Two.)

Joan's brain was injured immediately upon impact; she'd received bruises that could affect her cognitive, physical, and emotional abilities—but her problems might not stop there.

BRAIN STORMING

He was an outstanding hockey player. Some called him the best. But after seven years of hazy flashes, spots before his eyes, and dizziness caused by flying pucks, accurately aimed hockey sticks, and deadly tackles to the head, Lane MacDonald had had enough. "There was always the fear that by the end of the game, you might not be able to see very well," he told *Boston Globe* reporter John Power. "That was a tough thing to put yourself through." It was not even a year since he'd been named America's top college hockey player, but he simply decided that competitive hockey was not worth the risk of head injury. A player for Harvard, he hung up his skates in March 1990.

SECOND TO NONE

Unfortunately, the damage done by that ubiquitous blow could have some far-reaching implications. In addition to the initial damage done by the direct hit to Joan's skull, it was possible that she would suffer other damages, reverberating repercussions from the thud of that weapon on her skull. Often, these secondary problems would be seen within the first twenty-four hours of the trauma—if they occurred at all. And each of them would need an accurate diagnosis, constant medical surveillance, and possible surgery in order to prevent long-term damage.

These secondary brain injuries can include:

Bleeding

It's a fact. When you bruise your skin, you bleed—thanks to damaged blood vessels. The brain is no exception. But a scraped knee is easy to see and rectify. Unfortunately, a bleeding brain cannot be seen without the use of sophisticated diagnostic tools. To complicate matters even more, there are three different areas where bleeding can occur, each one capable of causing brain injury. If the blood vessels are hurt between the skull and the brain covering, it's called an *epidural hematoma*. If the bleeding occurs between the brain covering and the brain tissue itself, it's called a *subdural hematoma*. (For some reason, this is a popular "catch-all" diagnosis in many soap opera plots.) And if the blood vessels are damaged deep within the brain itself, it's called an *intracerebral hematoma*.

Swelling

It's a terrifying scenario: the blood compresses and damages brain tissue. The brain, in turn, expands with blood and fluid from the damaged areas. But there is no room for both the blood and the brain within the rigid confines of the skull. The brain begins to fill with pressure; it swells—with nowhere to go. This swelling, called *edema,* produces increased intracranial pressure and can only find space via....

Herniation

This is when the brain is literally squeezed out through a small opening in the base of the skull.

All of these conditions may require surgery, which is fraught with its own brand of danger. In order to stop bleeding or relieve pressure, a neurosurgeon, no matter how skilled, might damage additional surrounding tissue. Or she might decide to go with the better of two evils: removing brain tissue to stop a death-warrant-carrying infarction that can lead to enormous increases in intracranial pressure.

To help you understand how complex and dynamic these malfunctions can be, try this simple experiment. Dab a few drops of ink on a napkin. Notice how the drop begins to grow larger, spreading through the pattern of the nap-

kin, growing diffuse and fuzzy. Try it again. This time,
perhaps, the ink has remained pretty much in one spot.
This is exactly what can occur with brain damage. The
initial blow to the head has its own "dark blot" of problems.
But, within those first crucial 24 hours, that damage can
spread—affecting other areas throughout the brain. Or, as
in our second napkin/ink experiment, the damage might
stay put—and not radiate out to any other areas.

But there's another possibility. Say you did your ink
and napkin experiment on a tabletop, without putting any
protective paper underneath. The ink seeps through to the
table's beautiful oak veneer, ruining its finish with a river
of permanent blue. In "brain talk," this is called *epi-
phenomena*—and it means that damage in one area can
produce damage in completely different and faraway areas.
(See Chapter One.)

All these possibilities make it difficult to pinpoint the
problem areas involved in traumatic brain injury. But,
thanks to advances in technology, research, and diagnostic
tools, the job is getting easier.

Take Joan, for instance. She was lucky. She'd been
rushed to the emergency room of a hospital that knew what
it was doing; she'd also had a great deal of strength. She
was young, healthy, and fit. The tests showed only slight
damage; she didn't require surgery. Her brain swelling was
brought down with medication.

Joan's head injury and the trauma that led up to it
became a part of the past. Although she missed her first
six-month rotation, she is now in full swing, completing the
first year of residency. She has also installed an elaborate
alarm system in her apartment. And, yes, the newlyweds
have a dog who likes to bark at strangers.

LET'S GET PHYSICAL

Physical injury is one thing, but the physical impairments
they cause are another. Traumatic brain injury can cause a
variety of these symptoms. You or someone you know might
be suffering from one or more of them. Let's go over them
now:

Seizures

Major motor epilepsy, with full-blown convulsions, loss of consciousness, and writhing on the ground, is relatively rare following uncomplicated closed brain injury. Rather, because the fronto-temporal lobes are often involved in TBI, seizures may be more subtle. A patient might lose the passage of time. She might become spacey. He might make repetitive mouthing movements, over and over again. Although anticonvulsant medications may stop these seizures, they can also hinder alertness, attention, and memory. If a brain-injured person is already suffering from a cognitive impairment, this fact must be entered in the decision to medicate. Seizures are usually noticed within the first week of injury, but 5 percent of those injured will have them at a later date—and this number jumps to 15 percent in severely brain-injured patients.

Sensory Deficits

A woman who had been in a head-on collision came out fine—except that she could no longer smell anything. A man who'd fallen down the stairs could no longer hear out of one ear. Unfortunately, the loss of a sense is a common symptom after traumatic brain injury. This is not because a victim has lost an eye or an ear or a nose. Rather, the

---

BRAIN STORMING

Car Etiquette

"Buckle up, please" is more than manners. It's a matter of life and death. Studies have found that shoulder- and lap-type seat belts prevented injury in 50 to 65 percent of car accidents. In other words, between 12,000 and 16,000 lives are saved each year because of seat belts. And, just in case you thought your air bag was enough, here's some interesting news: Studies have shown that shoulder- and lap-type seat belts are better than air bags *alone* in preventing injuries.

So...definitely get your cars installed with air bags, but please, don't forget to buckle up as well!

sense-processing center in the brain has malfunctioned and the information that comes from this area cannot be assessed.

Loss of Motor Control and Coordination

It starts with brainstem damage. This leads to communication problems with the nerves connecting the brainstem with the neo-cortex and the cerebellum—the areas of the brain that control muscle movement and coordination. Disabilities can include:

- Weakness on one side of the body *(hemiplegia)*
- An inability to articulate words clearly—even though a patient's knowledge of language is intact. This is called *dysarthria.*
- Awkward gaits, an inability to coordinate muscle movements—these are all a part of what physicians call *ataxia.*
- Loss of dexterity—either in gross muscle movements, such as running and jumping, or in finely tuned motions, like playing the piano or knitting: incoordination.
- A lack of endurance during exercise—or even simply standing or sitting at rest is known as *adynamia.*

Fatigue

A study of mildly brain-injured patients found that feelings of irritability, fatigue, and anxiety *increase* after the injury—even as headaches and dizziness subside. This might not sound particularly bad, considering the other symptoms of brain injury, but think of it: head-injured people will need to sleep more. They'll need more breaks on the job. They'll tire easily after mental work or physical exercise. Here, sleep is not merely a "perchance to dream."

Decreased Tolerance for Drugs and Alcohol

John was in pain. His head injury made him feel confused, irritable. A drink always helped before. And if ever he needed one, it was now. But one drink and John had practically passed out. It's a difficult fact to absorb, but it's crucial for successful rehabilitation: brain injury affects the excitatory and/or depressing elements of drugs and alcohol. If alcohol makes you depressed, you'll be even more depressed. If you take cocaine, you'll be speeding at 180 m.p.h. Not only that, but the brain cells that malfunction from alcohol or drug abuse can ill afford to do so. After brain injury, you need all the proper functioning brain cells you have.

Headaches

It's the most common physical symptom—and, as studies have shown, headache pain, on the whole, happily decreases as the weeks go by. But if someone is suffering from post-concussive syndrome (See Part I), headaches may continue causing great discomfort even for those with mild brain injuries.

Confusion

A muddled thought. Disorientation. Forgetfulness. Aimless movements. Inappropriate actions. These are all elements of confusion, which is one symptom that can be pinpointed with *less* confusion than most. One study found that 93 percent of brain-injured patients who were confused had EEG abnormalities.

These are, very briefly, some of the physical impairments that can occur after traumatic brain injury. As difficult as they might sound to overcome, these disabilities are actually the easiest to work through and rehabilitate. Families, friends, and business colleagues are more accepting of someone who, say, comes to work in a wheelchair, who needs help cutting his meat at dinner, who needs more than eight hours of sleep—instead of someone who forgets to say thanks or acts irritable and childish.

The fact is that physical problems are easier to adjust to. Both the victims and their loved ones can adapt better. It is the intellectual impairments, the social and psychological inappropriateness, the loss of self, that in the long run create the most problems. These are the ones that are most difficult to accept, the most arduous to overcome for successful rehabilitation.

But difficult does not mean impossible. Acceptance and recovery can come with understanding. So, without further ado, let's go on to the cognitive and emotional deficits that can create such havoc and pain.

SEVEN

TBI: The Cognitive Factor

"I'm not stupid. I can add."

—Brian, 16 years old and moderately brain-injured

- Morgan was the king of real estate. He sold luxury
  houses as easily as another salesman would sell dis-
  count shoes. In fact, his company voted him "Best
  Salesman of the Year" three years in a row. But that
  was before his car accident—which left him with a
  broken leg, a few broken ribs, and a concussion. However, none of the neuroimaging studies he'd undergone
  showed any brain injury, and he was back on the job
  within four months, selling houses with the same pas-
  sion as before. But there was one crucial difference.
  Morgan talked a good game, but he'd lost the ability to
  follow through, to do his homework and plan. Consequently, he sold houses that had already been sold,
  that had city ordinance problems, that had not been
  properly appraised. Suit followed suit...and Morgan
  was out of a job. What no one—including Morgan—
  realized until it was too late was the fact that his
  so-called minor brain injury left him cognitively impaired.
- Joyce, 55, fell face-down down a flight of stairs—which
  damaged her frontal and temporal lobes. Today, in her
  rehabilitation center, she can tell you all about her
  high school prom, the dinners her mother prepared at

home, the wedding dress she wore. But she cannot tell what day it is—even if you list them first. Nor will she remember your name—or your face. She no longer can retain recent memories.

- Before he fell off his scaffold, Chris was a talented sculptor. He was an *enfant terrible,* temperamental and given to staring out his loft window for hours. In fact, he still looks deep in thought, his emotions in turmoil. But there's a difference. His tone, his emotions, his thoughts are all flat and empty. He has lost his verve and his imagination.

- Lynne had been an A student before she fell off her bicycle. She'd taken advanced courses and was college bound. Now, however, she has difficulty doing her multiplication tables without the aid of a calculator. She can't keep her history facts in order. Memorizing chemistry formulas remains a complete mystery. Unfortunately, Lynne's accident left her with learning disabilities. She needs a special school—and a change of future plans.

Different ages. Different lifestyles. Different points of view. But one thing these people all share is cognitive impairment—as a tragic result of traumatic brain injury. And, because our learning, memory, intelligence, and problem-solving skills are almost all located in the vulnerable fronto-temporal region of the brain, these cognitive deficits are more common than we might think.

BRAIN STORMING

The Chicken or the Egg?

Students who don't do well in school have been seen to be a new high-risk group for brain injury. A study of 80 head-injured patients who were doing poorly in school after their injury found that up to 50 percent of them also showed poor academic performance *before* their injury.

THE COGNITIVE EQUATION

A 1984 study found that the intellectual changes that occur in traumatic brain injury can hurt a patient's social rehabilitation—even if the changes are not noticed by others. And, because these changes can affect every aspect of a person's life, they must be noted, understood, and, ultimately, treated as best they can. These changes can be found in four main areas of cognitive impairment, four "Mind Matters" that can be affected by traumatic brain injury. Let's go over them now:

MIND MATTER #1: "Color My World Gray," or Impairments of Arousal

In order to be an active member of society, you have to interact with your environment. You need to have a degree of alertness, an ability to respond to stimuli—whether it's the perfume of the woman walking next to you or the smell of chicken roasting in the oven. But someone who has just injured his brain, who has come out of a lengthy coma, or who has had his brainstem or the sides of his frontal lobes injured may have changes in his level of alertness. He or she will be spacey—with a lethargic, "gray," flat view of the world. Like Chris, the sculptor in the above example, a person with arousal problems will be:

- Lethargic
- Inattentive
- Slow in reacting to and processing information
- Apt to drift off quickly when reading or thinking
- Unable to respond to any but the strongest stimuli (But strong doesn't necessarily mean important. An arousal impaired student might need to listen to his teacher's lecture on World War II for tomorrow's test, but he can only concentrate on the music coming from the "boom box" outside his window.)
- Slow in responding to others
- Prone to rambling conversations
- Inconsistent (If an arousal-impaired patient is in a very structured environment, he can perform tasks well—especially if given detailed, step-by-step instruc-

tions. But put this same person out in the real world, say, in an office where he's on his own, and his performance may drop drastically.

MIND MATTER #2: "Can't See the Forest for the Trees," or Attention and Concentration Deficits

A commuter misses the radio announcer's traffic update—even though he's been listening for it. A teen knows her school schedule, but she never seems to get to her class on time. A secretary never finishes his work for the day—even though he's skipped lunch and the work load is light. All these situations could be considered examples of attention deficits—and everyday frustrations for a brain-injured person.

But attention is a broad term. As with life, there's quantity—and there's quality. The *quality* of attention has to do with your ability to concentrate. When a person's attentional quality is impaired, he'll have trouble focusing in on a particular subject while ignoring background "noise." He can't be selective in his attention; he's too easily distracted—by the slightest interruption. Quality impairment can also mean there's a visual, auditory, or comprehension disability involved.

The *quantity* in your attention equation has to do with "attention span." A brain-injured person, as a rule, simply can't concentrate on a particular task or activity for as long a period as someone who is not attention impaired. She might ramble on when she speaks; she might change subjects in the midst of a conversation. He might have difficulty switching from one task to another—the way, for example, an administrative assistant stops typing to answer the phone without a second's thought.

Unfortunately, many neuropsychological tests consist of small, structured, and short tasks—which may mask these attention deficits. But when the attention-impaired person goes back on the job, to the long "workday" of changing routines, boring stretches of time, and stressful impromptu meetings, these problems will flare up with a frustrating vengeance.

BRAIN STORMING

A sampling of cognitive deficits that can occur after TBI:
- Memory difficulties
- Perceptual problems, including sight, sound, left/right orientation, and top/bottom orientation
- Neglect of one side of the body
- Lack of concentration
- Lack of initiation
- Inability to comprehend or understand a given situation or idea
- Expressive difficulties, including the inability to verbalize words or formulate thoughts
- Sequencing problems, with difficulty putting things in proper order
- Slowed responses—taking longer to do things
- Inflexibility (It's impossible to see a situation from any other point of view but your own. Your family might call this stubbornness)
- Disorganization
- Problem-solving difficulties
- An inability to deal with new learning situations

(From The HDI Coping Series #4: Life After Head Injury: Who Am I?, The Tampa General Rehabilitation Center, published by HDI Publishers, Houston, Texas.)

MIND MATTER #3: "The Buck Stops Here," or Executive Dysfunction

This is considered by many the cruelest blow of all. More than any other cognitive factor, executive functioning is at the heart of all our endeavors. It is the fuel that feeds the executive in the corner office. It is the spark that fires the writer in front of the word processor. It is the link that turns a concept into a reality for anyone, at any place, and in any walk of life. It involves the way we talk to people, deal with people, and carry out our daily lives.

Unfortunately, executive dysfunction is not easily discovered—or easily measured. Studies have found that brain-injured people with this impairment can do amazingly well on other cognitive tests. Why? Because executive functions deal with the *how* someone goes about his life—not what he knows or what he is intellectually capable of doing. Impairment here means "an organically based inability to plan, put into action, and carry through with an appropriate course of action."*

To add insult to injury, executive dysfunction is not only an all-pervasive tragedy, but it is a common result of even minor brain injury. Like other of the traits that contribute to our personality, executive functioning appears to be principally located in the vulnerable frontal region. But some of our planning functions are also located in other integrative brain structures, which can contribute to the executive dysfunction seen following severe injuries. In fact, it is such a difficult problem that studies have found that the dropout rate for patients with executive dysfunction in rehabilitation centers is 90 percent!

Its symptoms include:

- A lack of motivation. It often doesn't occur to an individual with executive dysfunction what the next thing is that he should do.
- Disorganization and poor planning.
- Empty promises. He lacks the needed self-awareness to make realistic promises.
- Difficulty attaining goals.
- Thoughtlessness and insensitivity to others.
- Unrealistic goal-setting. She cannot connect past failures with present plans.
- An inability to self-correct, self-evaluate, or self-regulate the work at hand.
- An inability to benefit from feedback from others—especially criticism.

Like the real estate salesman in this chapter's opening paragraph, a person suffering from executive dysfunction can "talk a good game" but be totally unable to follow through on any procedure. He may be the picture of

---

*Kay, Thomas, and Muriel Lezak, *Traumatic Brain Injury and Vocational Rehabilitation*.

BRAIN STORMING

Testing, Testing

Tinker Toys are not just for kids. They can also be used to show executive dysfunction. In a study done by Dr. Muriel D. Lezak, brain-injured patients who needed total support and supervision used less than 23 Tinker Toy pieces to build things. Those less severely injured used 23 or more pieces. But those in a control group who had no brain injury used all the 50 pieces that came in the kit.

More News: Those patients who had difficulty carrying out plans used few pieces—but they made items that were easily recognized. Those patients with problems in formulating goals used more Tinker Toy pieces—but the toy models they made were, on the whole, completely unrecognizable.

competence, responsibility, and apparent good judgment—but looks can be deceiving. He simply may not be able to put his plans into action. In fact, he may not be able to come up with that next idea; even the most obvious one. Period.

Here's an example: A man with stage fright spent weeks working on a speech, but he didn't think of taking his notes with him when he went to the podium. It wasn't an oversight or carelessness. It just didn't enter his mind that he'd need his notes.

Another example: A woman is set to go on a business trip. Her suitcase is packed and she's just asked the taxi driver to hurry to the airport. But when she rushes to the gate and the airline employee asks her for her ticket, she looks at him blankly. It didn't occur to her to bring her ticket.

And a few more: "Forgetting" to turn on an alarm clock to wake him up for work.... Not saying "thank you" when someone gives her a birthday present... "Forgetting" to call in sick when she can't get to work. Unfortunately, these behaviors are perceived by others as rudeness, laziness, and irresponsibility; they don't realize that it is often an organic problem, a result of brain injury that may or may not have been discovered at the time of the accident. The tragedy in all of this is that people who suffer from executive dysfunction will often lose their jobs and their friends—just when they need them the most.

MIND MATTER #4: "Memories are Made of This," or Memory and Learning Impairments

In *The Man Who Mistook His Wife for a Hat,* author Oliver Sacks quotes Luis Bunuel:

> You have to begin to lose your memory, if only in bits and pieces, to realize that memory is what makes our lives. Life without memory is no life at all.... Our memory is our coherence, our reason, our feeling, even our action. Without it, we are nothing....

Memory is crucial to who we are, but its loss is often a common after-effect of brain injury—sometimes temporary and sometimes long-lasting. An inability to remember events for a period of time *after* a brain injury is the most common memory impairment, but there are many others, as varied as memory itself.

- In *retrograde amnesia,* he will not remember the events leading up to the accident that caused his injury.
- In *post traumatic amnesia (PTA),* she will be confused for days or even months. She won't be able to remember day to day events *after* her injury. This often continues after a person has emerged from a coma and it is correlated with the amount of...
- *Residual deficits*—in functioning in which he may remember things only from the distant past because these memories are deeply ingrained. But he cannot store or retrieve new information. (He might also have a sensory impairment or an attention deficit which prevents him from responding to environmental cues that would normally "trigger" his memory.)
- *"Information in...information out."* Ask a person with a recent memory deficit to repeat what you just said

and she'll do so without great difficulty. But she'll forget what you said within minutes. She is only able to perform "immediate" recall, but there is no memory being consolidated or stored.

- *Incidental memory* problems include the inability to recall routine information. Forgetting where he put his keys...how to drive to a new part of town...when his next appointment takes place...all these examples of "absent-minded behavior" can be caused by brain injury.

- *Procedural memory* is the automatic pilot of memory, the deeply embedded habits and functions we perform without thought. This memory controls his bodily functions, his ability to eat, his knowledge of "cold" that enables him to pull the covers up when he goes to sleep. Usually this form of memory will remain intact after traumatic brain injury. The other form of memory which we are more accustomed to think of is...

- *Declarative memory*—and it's exactly how it sounds: her ability to explain how she drove somewhere, how she got dressed that morning, how she prepared her breakfast and what she actually ate. It's the lesson retained from school, those verbal exercises we heard our teachers say over and over again. It's language-based memory, the memory you'll have, say, as you read and learn from this book. Eventually, declarative memory will "hook" into a procedural routine. For example, once you've learned how to brush your teeth you don't think about each step as you perform this morning and evening ritual.

- *The learning link.* There is no way around it. When either form of the above memory become impaired, it will affect learning—which, in its most basic form, is committing new information to memory, integrating this knowledge/memory into our experiences, and using it as a frame of reference in our daily lives. Without memory, we cannot process and store information. Without the ability to process and store information, we cannot learn. Without an ability to learn, we can have no new memory....It's a vicious cycle that may include communication and language deficits—from an inability to express both verbal and written thoughts or comprehend what is being said to an inability to find words or understand printed material. These learning disabilities can all be caused by a brain injury—and all will affect our ability to process information.

MIND MATTERS

Memory loss. An inability to conceptualize or solve problems. A sensory deficit. Lack of insight or imagination. These "mind matters" add to the difficulties brain injured people have in adjusting to their injuries. They can also prevent solutions from being found—sabotaging many rehabilitation strategies that rely on these basic functions for their successful implementation. How? Through a patient's denying he has a problem to his making up facts to cover up his memory loss, from using his memory loss for extra attention or favors to feeling so angry and frustrated by the loss that he loses all motivation to get well.

There are many ways a good rehabilitation center can overcome these ultimately self-defeating behaviors—by providing encouragement, a safe, secure, prosthetic, learning environment, and step-by-step "chaining" strategies for building memories (especially procedural ones) back up—and we will review some of these strategies in Part III.

But for now, it's time to go on to the emotional and behavioral problems that can occur after brain injury. Some of them are a result of the cognitive and physical disabilities that occur at the time of the accident, but others are an indirect result of the injury itself. Let's go on to them now. . . .

EIGHT

TBI: The Psychosocial Factor

"I wish I could walk around with a sign that said, 'I am head-injured.'"

—Anonymous outpatient during a therapy session

I call Jill the "Urban Cowgirl" because every time she comes in to see me, she's wearing a rhinestone vest, red snakeskin boots with spurs, white jeans with studs, and an authentic heavyweight cowboy hat. This would be a smashing outfit if Jill was in the rodeo, or if I were the manager of a West Texas honky-tonk. However, these weekly meetings take place near downtown Houston, at my consulting office in the Texas Medical Center. Jill is an 18-year-old high school student and I'm her doctor.

Two years ago, Jill was involved in a car accident; she suffered a moderate brain injury that, unfortunately, caused both frontal and temporal lobe damage. Her disabilities during these two years included recent memory impairment and some left arm weakness. These deficits were being treated during her outpatient rehabilitation sessions; I was more concerned with her behavior, which showed a lack of self-awareness. She had a quick temper; she was extremely self-centered. Worse, she had a heightened sexuality; she flaunted herself in front of any boy she caught sight of—in class and out.

But Jill was completely unaware that she was turning people off. If anything, she couldn't understand why the boys at school snickered when she came walking up; she didn't know why the girls didn't want her on the soccer team anymore. She thought her "western" garb was great. It was cool, hip, and sexy. So why did everybody in the supermarket or the corner diner laugh at her when she walked in?

Like Jill's urban cowgirl dress, the psychosocial factors of TBI can have far-reaching implications, creating problems in school, on the job, and at home. The reasons why behavior is disturbed when the brain is injured are as varied as the way they are displayed—from Jill's rhinestone vest to, say, another person's long, unkempt hair....

"REALITY CHECK"

Sometimes inappropriate behavior is paradoxically the result of improving self-awareness—a depression or anger that springs up when you finally realize you are disabled, that you have lost the last three years of your life, that you can't walk without a cane, that you can't think of a word that's "on the tip of your tongue."

But sometimes behavioral problems are the result of deficits in self-awareness and impulse control, which may be caused by damage to "inhibiting" areas of the brain. When brain cells are damaged they release a whole host of chemicals that can create havoc in this intricately balanced system. Consequently, everything gets out of whack. With inhibiting neurotransmitters "out to lunch," the brain mushrooms into a wild, randomly impulsive machine—which translates into saying and doing embarrassing things, "wild" behavior, and even violence. Like the brakes in a car that need fluid, an injured brain can't stop short; it lacks a "braking mechanism." It's as if the brain is in rebellion—involved in a self-contained and very personal anarchy.

As Frederic R. Linge, a clinical psychologist and brain-injured individual, wrote in his inspiring article, "What Does It Feel Like to be Brain Damaged?":

I cannot cope with anger as well as I was able to do before my accident. Rage, related to my losses, does not lie just under the surface waiting to explode as it did earlier in my recovery. Yet, like any other person living in the real world, situations arise which make me justifiably angry, and I am still, today, slow to anger. The difference is that now, once I become angry, I find it impossible to 'put the brakes on' and I attribute this directly to my brain damage.*

THE PRIMARY LINK

If damage has been done to the temporal lobes, socially inappropriate behavior might come out during an electro-chemically mediated storm that medical professionals call *episodic dyscontrol syndrome (EDS)*. Here, the anger, and perhaps violence, will occur as a direct result of electrical dysfunction occuring within the brain. These episodes will start up suddenly and may be:

• Explosive, but undirected
• Dramatic
• Unpredictable and, mercifully,
• Brief

Sometimes episodic dyscontrol syndrome will not show up for months—or even years—after the accident. It may be triggered by a stressful situation, but, surprisingly, studies have found that EDS will not be triggered by looming, life-threatening traumas. It occurs with the trivial annoyances of life, the small stuff such as traffic, broken appointments, or burnt dinners.

THE SECONDARY LINK

When damage is done to the frontal lobes, the direct result of the injury is *not* always episodic emotional behavior—as it is with the temporal lobes' EDS. Here, the damage is done to the inhibiting neurotransmitters. It's felt that a deficit of these "messengers" helps set the stage for inappropriate behavior.

Nowhere is this situation more obvious than in the so called *frontal systems syndrome*. Here, the good news is that brain-injured patients manage to come through their accident with many of their "cognitive powers" intact. But the bad news is that their personalities go through tremendous changes—

*Reproduced with permission of the Minister of Supply and Services Canada 1991.

thanks to the injured anatomic structures and neurotransmitters that used to relay inhibiting behavioral messages like "Calm down" and "Not now." Symptoms may include:

- Lack of motivation
- Impaired social judgment
- Increased risk-taking
- A lack of regard for the future
- Substance abuse
- Failure to appreciate the effect of one's behavior on others
- Increased libido
- Poor grooming and daily hygiene
- Loudness
- Shallowness
- Indifference to the needs of others.

THE THINKING MAN'S ANGST

In patients with frontal systems deficits, inappropriate behavior occurs *despite* "cognitive ability." Psychosocial problems may also occur despite the absence of severe "cognitive deficits." Self-regulation, including the ability to know right behavior from wrong, to act in a mature manner, to summon up self-control, is another component of executive functioning—just like goal-setting, planning, thinking, and taking initiative. Thus, psychosocial disturbances can be a direct result of a brain-injured person's executive dysfunction. Without an ability to think conceptually, there can be no analysis of a given situation. Without this analysis, there is just the impulse to act.

NO, PLEASE, AND THANK YOU

Manners are taught. So is appropriate social behavior. By the time a reasonably normal person is an adolescent, the rules and mores of a society have been in place, ingrained, and in sync with the rest of the world. But brain injury can destroy all that we know about saying "Thank you," playing with the Jell-O, forgetting to use a knife and fork, or leaving our pants unzipped in public.

What makes things worse is the fact that often brain-injured people aren't even aware that they're not acting correctly. Throwing the Jell-O across the room when they're frustrated or angry feels just fine, thank you. Ditto for the lamp, the chair—or the orderly. But it's important not to take this aggression personally. In the same way they aren't always aware of incorrect behavior, they usually don't harbor any resentment once the flare-up has subsided.

But psychosocial problems can try one's patience. Some of the more off-putting behaviors in brain-injured persons are....

THE BIRDS AND THE BEES, OR: SEXUAL PROBLEMS

Studies have found that 50 percent or more of TBI persons have sexual disturbances—but these studies are based on research done only on those behaviors that are displayed in rehabilitation wards. In actuality, medical professionals today believe that some degree of sexual dysfunction is universal among brain-injured people. In fact, it's one the reasons there are so many divorces in families following TBIs.

BRAIN STORMING

Sex Myths and the Disabled

1. The disabled are asexual. They can't feel sexy or have sexual feelings because they are handicapped.
2. The disabled cannot have sex. Because of the handicap, a disabled person is unable to function sexually.
3. The disabled participate in abnormal sex. After all, the handicap is abnormal, so the sexual activities they perform must be so, too.

All these are myths—which a brain-injured person will encounter in the real world. Family and friends must be aware of them—and prevent them from becoming a reality.

Damaged frontal and temporal lobe structures are not the only culprits here. Sexual dysfunction can also be caused by damage done to the hypothalamus, which regulates our sexual drive. Imbalances here can result in either abnormally high sexual drive or an extremely low one. Sexual dysfunction is not just a problem in the bedroom. It can hinder a brain-injured person's re-entry into the community. When a man with TBI, for example, acts sexually aggressive in a singles bar, it will result in a lot of "get lost" remarks—to say the least. A brain-injured woman, on the other hand, can become "easy prey" because of her poor impulse control, impaired judgment, and low self-esteem. Aggressor or victim, both roles bring rejection and pain to the brain-injured person—and with that rejection comes even lower self-esteem.

But there's more. Many brain-injured people have problems with perception—and that includes self-perception. They are not aware of how they look; unkempt hair, wrinkled clothes, and dirty nails can all go unrecognized to them. Like the Urban Cowgirl, they just can't understand why no one will give them a second look.

On a more personal note, sexual dysfunction in a brain-damaged spouse is usually coupled with role reversal and personality changes that dramatically alter "old" more comfortable behavioral patterns. Thus, intimate sexual relationships are drastically changed; couples are easily alienated.

Here's an example: One brain-injured patient, a man, had a heightened sexual drive—coupled with a short-term memory loss. Several months after he'd been discharged from his rehabilitation center, during a consultation with me regarding his behavior, his wife could no longer hold back the tears. Her husband not only wanted sex all the time, but he'd forget that he'd had sex soon after they'd had relations. Consequently, he "kept after" his wife all the time....

I SEE RED, OR: ANGER AND INAPPROPRIATE AGGRESSIVENESS

A fact: 80 percent of prisoners jailed for violence have temporal lobe abnormalities. Another fact: Agitation and aggressiveness are commonly seen in TBI during the early stages of rehabilitation. As the inspiring Frederic R. Linge also writes in "What Does It Feel Like to be Brain Damaged?":

> As the profound coma lifted towards the end of the first week...I showed a great deal of agitation and rage. Frequently, I would fight desperately to be free of the traction and would hit out angrily at those around me...My family recalls that I seemed quite desperate to communicate and my failure to do so infuriated me as much as the physical immobility.*

This makes sense. The confusion in those early days of emerging from coma, combined with the alien surroundings of the hospital ward would make anyone lash out. Think of it: you've had this severe accident that, chances are, you won't recall—ever. Suddenly, you awake from this very deep sleep, unable to move, unable to speak, in pain, and in a strange place....

Frequently, in these early days of recovery, a brain-injured person will hallucinate. (Fredric R. Linge imagined himself on an ocean liner with his wife; his hospital windows were portholes.)

Finally, as the coma recedes, as the hallucinations pass, and as rehabilitation begins, a general feeling of irritability moves in. This anger and frustration can settle in for just a few days—or several months. Yes, it's true. This new-found, injury-induced agitation will often be in control before the year is out. But the aggression can also have a life of its own, occasionally surviving for a much longer period of time as a *learned* response to stress— coming into play whenever social, financial, or personal problems rear their heads.

The anger and frustration will reach their heights as disabilities become more and more apparent, as awareness of one's limitations increases. Indeed, reality can be so difficult, so compromised, organically as well as psychologically, that one study found that 40 percent of brain-injured people "refused" or were unable to admit their disabilities seven years later! As Frederic Linge says:

> For many weeks, I denied that I had lost my sense of taste and smell. I never mentioned the loss to

*Reproduced with permission of the Minister of Supply and Services Canada 1991.

anyone while I was in the hospital and it was only on the "safe ground" of home that I took the first steps towards admission of this deficit. This was to complain to my wife that food "tasted funny." I accused her of having added something strange to it; then I theorized that she had bought food that wasn't fresh or that had gone bad. Finally, when I was able to accompany her to the store, buy the food myself and be assured of its quality, and do the actual cooking myself, I had to admit that the fault was not in the food itself but in my own senses.*

But whether a result of dysregulated neurotransmitters caused by bruised temporal lobes, or as a result of recognizing a painful reality, the anger hurts. Period. Unfortunately, this anger is usually directed at those closest to the brain-injured person: his family, his friends, his therapists, his rehabilitation team. And, even more unfortunately, this anger can quickly turn to physical aggression—which translates into destroyed property or a direct hit to someone's person. One patient of ours exploded when a peer changed the channel on the TV; our patient attempted to hit him.

At least this aggressive act was committed within the confines of a hospital. What if this same patient had been at a store, growing angrier and angrier at a salesperson because she wouldn't check him out of the store fast enough! The salesperson wouldn't know that her customer had had a TBI. She'd just see someone unruly. She would try to explain that she was working as fast as she could, but he would be too embarrassed to say he didn't know how to count his money. He'd grow more frustrated and angry, becoming more and more certain that the salesperson was testing him, taunting him. He might strike out—at her. The next thing you know he's in big trouble...

This is only an imaginary scenario, but it happens more frequently than you might imagine. I have had several patients who are at the Neurobehavioral Institute of Houston because they came within a hairbreadth of shooting someone. One boy almost killed his mother. One man almost shot his wife. One woman destroyed her house. The aggression marches on....

One more point: This anger is closely related to lack of impulse control. It's truly "acting without thinking" be-

*Reproduced with permission of the Minister of Supply and Services Canada 1991.

cause the mechanisms that allow us to conceptualize, to analyze, to realize the consequences of our deeds, are not working right. Add to this the extreme emotional ups and downs due to damage in the limbic system and you have a person who is indeed out of control—often by no fault of his own.

Sad, yes. Painful, yes. In fact, one emotion that frequently comes to roost in a brain-injured person is...

COLOR MY WORLD BLUE, OR: DEPRESSION

I remember periods of intense depression during which I would retreat to the bedroom for hours on end, covering up my true feelings by saying to myself that 'the noise of the children was too much for me.'*

This is Frederic R. Linge talking again, and it makes sense. The denial, the pain, the general loss of self-esteem, the disorientation... all can make a person depressed.

BRAIN STORMING

Up from Depression

Studies have found that depression is extremely common in severely brain-injured people between three and six months after their trauma. But the good news is that it usually doesn't last, especially when correctly treated.

Depression is partly, after all, anger turned inward. It is the despair behind the frustration of being brain-injured. As one of my patients said, "It wasn't my fault. I didn't ask to be brain-injured."

Depression is abetted further by the rejection that occurs because the brain injured survivor is "different." Combine this with the lack of attention to personal grooming habits, and you'll see people running away in droves. Rejection settles in to stay. Friends lose their patience and move

*Reproduced with permission of the Minister of Supply and Services Canada 1991.

on to other things. Families, unable to hide their own unhappiness and impatience, stop coming by to visit. Jobs are lost—or never found. One study found that of 864 brain-injured Americans, only 75 percent had found jobs even fifteen years after their accidents!

The only way to cope for some brain-injured people is with alcohol, drugs, or more inappropriate attention-seeking behavior. But these methods are self-destructive and result in more loss of self-esteem. It can become a vicious cycle with no end in sight.

In fact, studies have found that psychosocial problems will not go away by themselves. Therapy is needed. When the indefatigable Mr. Linge finally went into his therapist's office and cried, he began the long road back. When Jill, the Urban Cowgirl, gradually began to learn that her costume looked "funny" through various techniques I used in my therapy sessions (see Chapter Eleven), she began to change her behavior.

Therapy can help.

I AM A ROCK, OR: ADYNAMIA

Think the opposite of aggression and you'll understand adynamia. Because of the way the brain has been damaged, an adynamic person will lack initiative. He may actually possess the desire to get a job, to find a date for Saturday night, to even do something as simple as join in the game of charades in the hospital lounge—but he doesn't. He simply lacks the interest and the energy.

She's confused; she can't perceive or conceptualize a specific situation.

He feels overwhelmed.

She finds it impossible to begin rewarding social, community, and career-oriented activities.

He becomes isolated, lonely, and even more depressed—relying on others much too much for structure and meaning in his life.

She becomes too dependent.

In his book *The Effects of Brain Damage on the Personality in Psychiatry*, Kurt Goldstein describes a patient "who never seemed to be concerned about his family. He never spoke of his wife or children and was unresponsive when we questioned him about them. When we suggested to him that he should write to his family, he was utterly indifferent. He appeared to lack all feelings in this respect...But while he was at home, he conducted himself in the same way that any man would in the bosom of his family. He was kind and affectionate to his wife and children and interested in their affairs insofar as his abilities would permit. Upon his return to the hospital from such a visit, he would smile in an embarrassed way and give evasive answers when he was asked about his family; he seemed utterly estranged from his home situation...His behavior was the result of the fact that he could not summon up the home situation when he was not actually there."

This man was completely incapable of thinking about his family when he wasn't with them. He couldn't get into a car and drive to see them. Nor could he pick up a phone and call. Love is one thing, but initiating action is another.

But there is one more TBI factor that still must be mentioned. It is the culmination of all these physical, cognitive, and psychosocial deficits. It is the changed personality, the "alien self," the most elusive and the most critical factor of all.

NINE

TBI AND THE ALIENATION OF SELF

"Self is the only prison that can ever bind the soul."

—*The Prison and the Angel,*
Henry Van Dyke (1852–1933)

"He's a different person."

"I don't know...I can't explain it. But she's not the same anymore. It's subtle."

"My body's fine, but my soul is lost."

"I'm still me. But I'm not."

"No one has to tell me now. I realize I've forever changed."

"This isn't my husband."

"What happened to my child?"

"All my friends are gone."

"I have to try harder now."

Family members. Friends and lovers. Brain-injured patients themselves. I've heard these words over and over again. And, even now, after years of practicing medicine, it is these statements of selfhood that strike the cruelest blow.

If an adult becomes blind, it is indeed a tragedy. But, after a period of rehabilitation, of denial, anger, and depression, he will learn to cope with his disability. His mind will help him discover new ways of living; he can teach himself self-sufficiency and organization. In time, his blindness will usually be accepted. Although he can no longer see the way he did, he will still be himself; he will still have the same tastes, the same dreams, the same beliefs. His essence or, as the poets say, his soul, will still be intact.

But suppose this man had been brain-injured. The very organ that would help him cope with his disability is injured! Like the Urban Cowgirl who could not see that her dress was inappropriate, a brain-injured person is often not aware of his disability—at least at first. On one level, this is a blessing. Unlike the blind person, he is free from the pain of knowing he is "lost." But this lack of self-awareness causes a whole host of other problems—and gives rehabilitation its greatest challenge.

THE ALIEN AMONG US

From neurologists to psychiatrists, from scientists to behaviorists—each field of medicine has its own beliefs and its own set of assumptions. But no matter the amount of research, the countless studies, the carefully tabulated results, all of us intuitively know that an electrochemical reaction or a genetic predisposition does not define "personhood" and finally falls short; still missing is something that can't be explained.

There is a part of us that no one sees, yet everyone who cares about us knows. It's not behavior. It's not a chemical reaction. It is the self. And it is this essence that makes us individuals, that gives us a personality, a temperament. When someone is brain-injured, that personality, along with other functions of our brain, will be disrupted—and, in the same way a person will lose his memory, or become confused, or forget your name, you will also see changes in who that person is.

From *The Invasion of the Body Snatchers* to *1984,* the loss of one's self has always been seen as the supreme violation, the stuff of science-fiction nightmares and political polemics.

It is no wonder that this alien self is so difficult to understand and work with—and why it poses such problems for a brain-injured patient's family and friends.

The ultimate alien self comes from Oliver Sacks' book *The Man Who Mistook His Wife for a Hat,* in which he

BRAIN STORMING

Although traumatic brain injury can cause families to separate and marriages to fail, in some cases, it's viewed as a blessing. Take the case of the 62-year-old salesman who had a drinking problem. He fell while intoxicated and suffered a severe closed brain injury.

Now, before his accident, he was always out carousing. He was abusive to his wife; he was slovenly; he was often drunk and angry. Unfortunately, after his accident, he could not return to work—but that didn't disturb his wife.

The brain injury also lowered his desire for carousing—and he stopped drinking all together. He became positively cheerful and humorous. He might not have remembered much, but he stayed home. He was no longer abusive or cranky. His wife knew where he was at all times—and she enjoyed his jokes. She was actually pleased!

Adapted from "The Psychiatry of Closed Head Injury" by Michael Bond, in *Psychological, Social, and Family Consequences*, Oxford, England: Oxford University Press, 1984.

describes a certain Mrs. B, a one-time research chemist, who had developed a brain tumor. As the tumor grew and changed, so did her personality. She become "hyper," full of wisecracks and sarcasm. On one occasion she called Dr. Sacks "Father," because he reminded her of a priest. On another occasion, she called him "Sister," because of his white uniform. Other times, she called him "Doctor" because of his stethoscope. To her, it meant no difference. In fact, she says, as Dr. Sacks writes:

"'But they mean nothing to me. They're no different for *me*. Hands...Doctors...Sisters...' she added, seeing my puzzlement. 'Don't you understand? They mean nothing—nothing to me. *Nothing means anything*...at least to me.'"

Dr. Sacks was shocked; he continued to question her. He wondered if this way of thinking bothered her.

It didn't. He continues:

"Was this denial? Was this a brave show? Was this the 'cover' of some unbearable emotion? Her face bore no deeper expression whatever. Her world had been voided of feeling and meaning. Nothing any longer felt 'real' (or 'unreal'). Everything was now 'equivalent' or 'equal'—the whole world reduced to a facetious insignificance....

"Mrs. B, though talkative and intelligent, was somehow not present—'de-souled'—as a person."

Mrs. B's case was truly extreme. Her self had become completely alien—and perhaps no amount of rehabilitation would have helped.

In many brain-injured people following acceleration/deceleration injuries, their ability to be self-reflective is lost. Along with executive functioning, our self-reflective function is felt to be a function of the "frontal systems." When this area gets damaged, so does our self-awareness, our ability to have insight into our problems—and our knowledge of how we've changed.

Take Jill, the Urban Cowgirl. In her mind, her rhinestone vest was gorgeous. She didn't see her protruding stomach, her dirty hair, her oversized snakeskin boots. What Jill was thinking was that Dr. Cassidy's the jerk, or her parents, or her friends. Why? Because we kept saying that something was wrong—and she just didn't see it. Her mother would say, "Take a shower! Comb your hair!" Her sister gradually withdrew and spent less and less time at home. Her father would ask her to come to the dinner table properly washed and dressed....

But Jill didn't know what they were talking about. Her brain was saying, "What's going on here? I don't think what you're saying is true. I think I look great!"

Unfortunately, the more Jill acted the Urban Cowgirl role, the more she alienated her family and her friends. She became more and more isolated—without understanding why no one cared about her anymore.

Like other brain-injured people whose self-reflective functions are injured, Jill's inherent problems with her TBI would have escalated—if she hadn't received quality care. The confusion, the inability to concentrate, to focus or plan, would snowball. The anger would become even more heated. Resentments would build. Disabilities would become handicaps. Reality and its acceptance would fade even further and further away. Depression would mushroom—ending perhaps in isolation... or self-inflicted death.

Unfortunately, this is a too common scenario. A study of 25 severely head-injured patients found that all of them believed they had changed substantially since they had their accident—but they were also confident that they would return to their old selves within a year! This attitude might protect a patient from an onslaught of pain in the beginning of his rehabilitation, but, in the long run, it will only hamper successful recovery. Step by step, here's the deadly process, adapted from *Life After Head Injury: Who Am I?* (The HDI Coping Series #4, by the Tampa General Rehabilitation Center):

THE DEADLY CYCLE

1. The accident occurs.
2. A person's head is injured, resulting in...
3. Cognitive problems, such as memory loss and decreased concentration...
4. Physical problems, such as motor impairments and headaches...
5. Psychosocial problems, such as anger and depression, impulsivity and inappropriate violence. These problems, in turn, result in...
6. A sense of alienation, a loss of self.
7. With this loss of self comes more loss: friends, family, job, school grades, hobbies and activities.
8. All of which creates: decreased intimacy, decreased productivity, decreased enjoyment, decreased life satisfaction...
9. And more cognitive, psychosocial, and physical problems.

But it doesn't have to be this way.

THE CYCLE OF LIFE

It's called effective rehabilitation—and it can work. In addition to cognitive, physical, and psychosocial therapies, a good rehabilitation program takes into special account the alien self. Rather than try to help a patient recover his old sense of self, studies have shown that a good rehab center helps the survivor accept his *new* self.

Of course, this is no simple task. People have developed their sense of self over the years. Their environment, their motivations, their beliefs, their circle of friends—all stem from this developed and refined sense of self. Then boom! A tragedy. A traumatic head injury occurs and this old, comfortable self is forever gone.

But, believe it or not, this fact can be accepted—and brain-injured patients can grow to understand and even like who they are today. They can be literally "reborn."

For Jill, the Urban Cowgirl, this meant months and months of showing her that other people's perceptions were valid, too. I brought countless photographs into our therapy sessions that showed her, in black and white and sometimes color, what she had looked like before the accident. I asked some of her old friends to come in; I pointed out that they were dressed differently than she. We videotaped several sessions and watched the playback together as we discussed that new person depicted on the video. Slowly, after many sessions, many visual aids, Jill began to understand. She realized that, perhaps, these people who were a part of her world had valid feelings, too.

This struggle to accept a new self is a focal point of our rehabilitation program at the Neurobehavioral Institute in Houston, and I'll discuss this process in more depth in Chapter Eleven.

It's a fact: if you are significantly brain-injured, you will never be exactly the same person again. Period. But you can learn to *accept* that you are not this same person. And you can have dignity and meaning in your life. It will be a different life—but it can still be a meaningful one.

Incidentally, Jill is now wearing Gap jeans and simple sneakers. She's discovered a talent for music and she's learning to play the guitar. And she does volunteer work part-time at a local nursing home.

This is it. The damage has been done and discussed. It's now time to talk to returning, of rehabilitation that works, of life after TBI.

Life is waiting.

PART III

RETURNING

TEN

Four Factors That Can Help Rehabilitation Success

"I believe I can do anything. But I know I can't."

—Brain-injured patient at the
Neurobehavioral Institute of Houston

In 1983, Billy fell down a flight of stairs and hit his head. Although he was a bit wobbly, he didn't think too much about it. He wasn't bleeding; there were no bumps or bruises. In fact, he was more concerned about his broken wrist, which was causing him a great deal of pain.

His wrist healed; Billy went on about his life. He was making a good salary as a construction worker. He'd just bought a modest house in a quiet neighborhood, and his wife and two kids seemed happy.

All was well for the next week. But when Friday night rolled around, everything changed. Billy and a few of the guys went out for a beer before going home. He drank one beer and felt dizzy—almost as if he'd already had several beers. But he ordered another one; he kept up with the guys. Suddenly the room began to spin around. Billy began to raise his voice. He made a fist... and that's the last thing he remembered until he woke the next morning in bed. His nose was swollen and crusted with blood; his wrist throbbed and his stomach hurt. Apparently Billy had gotten into a fight.

But that was only the beginning. Billy began to get angry at the drop of a hat—and not just after a few drinks.

He screamed at his wife and kids. He punched a hole in a wall. He kicked open the locked bedroom door and hit his wife.

That was the last straw. Billy's wife left with the children. She filed for divorce.

Billy became even more upset. He lost his job and his house. He turned to drugs, specifically marijuana and cocaine, to ease his pain.

Finally, Billy entered a drug abuse program at the local hospital in 1986. His speech was slurred, his memory was poor, and he could barely walk. It wasn't until then—a full three years after his accident—that his closed head injury was diagnosed. Now, he not only had to deal with the psychological problems he incurred *after* his injury—but the brain injury deficits themselves. It was a double dose of reality for Billy.

All in all, this would sound like a "sad sack" story, a lesson in prevention. But there's more here than meets the eye.

First of all, Billy had *always* been a fighter. He'd come home drunk more Friday nights than he could count. He also loved to drink; it just took more mugs of beer to reach his "fighting stance" *before* the accident.

In fact, Billy had been a wild risk-taker all his life. He drove fast, played fast, and dreamed impractical "get rich" dreams. Perhaps, his wife would have left him anyway—and he'd already been warned on the job more than once.

Take all these elements together and you have a person with a high risk of getting a head injury. Unfortunately, a high risk for brain injury also means additional complications that may preclude successful rehabilitation if an accident occurs.

Although there is no set formula or predisposition etched in stone, there are six characteristics that can aid or hinder recovery, six "Head Gears" that can equip someone for rehabilitation failure—or success.

HEAD GEAR #1: SEVERITY OF INJURY

The length of coma. The amount of amnesia after the injury. The extent of initial brain damage and the subsequent neurologic complications. All of these are factors in determining the severity of injury—and affect the chances of successful rehabilitation.

Comas are not an everyday occurrence. If a person goes into one, it makes sense that there's been brain injury. The same holds true for what doctors call post-traumatic amnesia—the empty pockets of memory following the accident. The more this amnesia lingers, the more likely brain damage has been extensive. Here's proof: A 1988 study found conclusive evidence that there was a correlation between the length of a coma and the length of a patient's stay in a rehabilitation center.

BRAIN STORMING

The Glasgow Coma Scale is used to measure the depth of a coma, which, in turn, is one indicator of the severity of injury. Eye opening, motor and verbal response to, say, a prick of a needle are noted on a graduated scale.

A low score of 3–4 means that the coma is very "deep"—and the patient has not opened his eyes, moved a muscle, or spoken.

The highest score is 15, which means that a patient's eyes have opened and his pupils are reacting normally to light. He has heard and obeyed a command; he can answer questions. He can also normally move his extremities at request.

Anything below a score of 8 is considered *true* coma, and is indicative of severe "injury."

Age also has an effect on outcome. Studies have found that young adults who wake from a coma return to work at a higher rate than older people.

Epilepsy, too, is a "severity of injury" factor. If a patient suffers from repeated, late occurring seizures, it can mean that the damage done to the brain is extensive—and rehabilitation will be that much harder.

A close relative to epilepsy is agitation. A study found that a patient's agitation during the early stages of injury will have a direct bearing on the amount of behavioral disturbances he will ultimately have. The more agitation, the more disturbance.

But, after all is said and done, it's important to remember that this "head gear" deals only with probability. Throughout this book, you have seen cases of mild brain injury that have led to a long-term concussive syndrome. You have also seen that seemingly minor bumps on the head create damage in the fronto-temporal lobes of the brain, without the victim being unconscious for more than a few minutes at most!

HEAD GEAR #2: PRE-TRAUMA FACTORS

It's called survival of the fittest. Individuals who are healthier, mentally and emotionally, will have a better chance of a successful rehabilitation. Studies have found that the more intelligent a person is, the more capable she is in finding ways to cope with her cognitive disabilities, to discover ways of circumventing her problems.

Highly motivated survivors, too, have a better chance of "making it." Personalities do go through a transformation after a head injury, but dominant characteristics shine through: people who respond well to challenges, who are self-motivated, who are stubborn and tenacious and refuse to give in to their pain can do well—especially if, at the same time, they are open to others, ready and willing to receive their help and support.

This character sketch is not an idealized work of fiction. Nor is it a portrait of an obsessive perfectionist. This type of person might be highly motivated, but he may also be "unrealistic." If he sets too high a goal for himself, he may set himself up for difficulties in accepting his new limitations in life.

No, this sketch is one of realistic strength. People with this temperament will automatically have high self-esteem—which, as with most things in life, will help them struggle through the frustrations of rehabilitation.

On the other side of the coin, there are people like Billy, people who had personality problems *before* their injury occurred that will definitely complicate their rehabilitation. Some of these "negative" personality traits are a history of depression or substance abuse, paranoia, feeling overwhelmed in times of stress, and resisting help when it is offered.

HEAD GEAR #3: A FAMILY AFFAIR

Brain injury doesn't just happen to one person. When a loved one is hurt, the whole family is affected. Guilt...anguish...frustration...sadness...denial—everyone in the victim's sphere will feel the reverberations of that traumatic brain injury. But family support is crucial. A family who understands, who goes through the process with their loved one, who is patient and kind, can only help. But this is easier said than done—especially when everyone is going through such turmoil themselves. In fact, at times, it is simply an impossibility to be there for the injured family member. But it will leave its mark: A study done of 39 severely brain-injured patients and 35 of their "significant others" found that the lack of a close, sharing, and confiding relationship had a direct correlation to any emotional disorders the patients ultimately had.

A complicated situation, yes. But not an impossible one. Because family issues are so dynamic and complex, I've devoted an entire chapter to them. (See Chapter Twelve.)

HEAD GEAR #4: THE "REALITY" FACTOR

Standard equipment for successful rehabilitation includes the capacity for the brain-injured person to:

Become Aware of Deficits

At the Braintree Hospital Eighth Annual Traumatic Head Injury Conference on October 14, 1987, David E. Walker presented his research on the prediction of recovery for closed head-injured adults. His results? Patients who denied their problems, who refused to acknowledge their limitations, and who made elaborate excuses whenever these limitations reared their embarrassing heads had a poor chance of recovery. Further, this denial is usually combined with socially inappropriate behavior—further hindering the chances for successful rehabilitation.

Accept the Reality of a New Self

Study after study has shown that successful rehabilitation can only occur if therapists and physicians help patients adapt to their *new* self—rather than promote the possibilities of returning to their old ones. It usually can't happen and it just postpones the inevitable—creating anger, frustration, and depression.

Set and Accept New Goals

We have seen many examples of brain-injured persons who have become frustrated in their attempts to get back their old jobs or old lives. One of my patients, a vice-president in a consulting firm, wanted to be a vice-president again—even though he was no longer capable of adequately performing this role. He kept "banging" his head against countless office doors...he began to drink. Finally, he accepted his new limitations and found another career in marketing.

Another example: Charlie was left paraplegic and unable to walk alone when his brain stem was severely injured in a motorcycle accident. Because of his disability he refused to resume dating again (or to go much of anywhere

---

BRAIN STORMING

Ride With the Wind

As reported in *The New York Times*: In 1975, when 47 states passed a law requiring that all motorcycle drivers wear helmets, fatalities dropped by half. But when 27 states subsequently repealed this law, fatality rates *rose* 45 percent.

As researched by General Motors Laboratories: Motorcycle deaths increased in those states that repealed their helmet law—in 24 cases out of 26.

The statistics are staggering. Why take a chance? A motorcycle helmet not only can mean the difference between life and death—but the difference between a *full* life and a brain-injured one. Think about it.

for that matter) until he could walk "normally" again. Well, it could take years. In fact, it might never happen. Charlie has to live life now. At 19, he has a whole world ahead of him—and we at the Neurobehavioral Institute of Houston are showing him how to accept himself and begin anew.

This "head gear" presents a challenge for physicians and therapists. Because problems with executive functioning and memory may limit a patient's ability to set and accept new goals, a therapist must repeat things over and over again, becoming almost like an "external frontal lobe," to get the message across that:

1. The patient is different from who he once was, and...
2. She is, like the Urban Cowgirl, *unaware* that she is different.

Once the new self is integrated into a patient's psyche, once he fully understands and believes that he has changed, successful rehabilitation can occur. (I'll be going into this rehabilitation process in more detail in the next chapter.)

HEAD GEAR #5: FINANCIAL SUPPORT

Although most of us are uncomfortable discussing the financial realities that accompany any catastrophic illness or accident, we need to address them up front and head on. Despite taking quite a beating in the popular press and on Capitol Hill, the American health-care system remains the world's finest. This is especially true of our neurotrauma care. Within the last two decades, we've begun saving thousands of lives that once would have been lost. However, these advances have not been cheaply won; they are expensive from both a labor and technology perspective.

Since we cannot "cure" brain injury the way we do say, strep throat, treatment requires massive support systems that sustain life and limit further complications—while mind and body heal over time. Those old enough to remember the polio epidemic are well aware of this: Huge iron

BRAIN STORMING

The Matter of Cost

- A study of 487 brain-injured patients between the ages of 16 and 45 found that the cost for a mild traumatic injury in one year cost approximately $8100. Those with severe injuries incurred costs up to $105,350.
- The cost for all people between the ages of 16 and 45 in Maryland hospitals for treatment of trauma cost approximately $109 million in 1983.
- The average cost per day at the Mississippi Methodist Rehabilitation Center, a typical rehab center, is $725.00. If a head-injured person needs respiratory care, the cost becomes $870.00.

With brain injuries becoming the "silent epidemic" of the nineties, we must find ways to help finance these costs—and adjust our insurance and government policies.

lungs "breathed" for desperately ill and paralyzed victims while the ravages of the virus ran their course. Expensive, yes, but this supportive technology provided the only hope available at the time. However, research in the basic medical sciences continued and a preventive vaccine was discovered. Millions of lives have been saved and the cost of "polio" is virtually nonexistent today. We have similar hopes for the research currently being done with various pharmacologic agents by those scientists who study experimental brain injury.

Headway is being made, but we're still years away from a "cure." For now, we all must shoulder the costs of expensive supportive treatments—because they may provide the only hope for one of our loved ones or ourselves.

This is not to say that the costs of adequate care can be easily borne: A survey sent out to 100 parents and 50 spouses of brain-injured patients found that the average length of stay for acute care was 49 days—at a cost of approximately $60,000. Doctor and hospital bills added up to a staggering $92,811.70. Drugs and other medical expenses averaged over $11,000. Legal expenses were over $30,000. Modifications done on the home to create a better environment for the brain-injured person was over $3,000. Speech, physical therapy and other specialized therapies came to about $15,000.

With costs like these, it wasn't surprising that many of those surveyed responded that their brain-injured loved ones needed help—but they weren't getting it. Others wrote that they had to borrow money or go bankrupt to pay their bills. Still others got second jobs—or re-entered the work force.

Of course, legal damages, worker's compensation, and other health insurances help foot the bills, but the results of this survey still showed that the costs of brain injury can be overwhelming for many families.

Nonetheless, a good, solid "umbrella" health insurance policy offers some peace of mind. And it will help insure that a patient gets adequate care.

HEAD GEAR #6: THE WORKPLACE AND THE COMMUNITY ENVIRONMENT

The opportunity to perform meaningful work is a critical element for emotional well-being in all of us. Brain-injured patients are no exception. When they are about to re-enter the work force, they need to find jobs that will help their self-esteem—by providing a necessary forum to demonstrate competence and enable them to experience a series of small successes. They need jobs that can be flexible, where employers understand their limitations—and are willing to work with them. The availability of such a job and such a boss is crucial for vocational re-entry. Remember Frederick R. Linge, the brain-injured man whose words were so inspiring in the preceding chapters? After he'd gone through much rehabilitation, after he had suffered through much anguish, self-examination, and determination, he re-entered the work force as a clinical psychologist—the job he held before his accident.

A community, too, can help a survivor's re-entry by supporting local programs designed to bridge the gap between hospital and home. Community-based head-injury programs, family support groups, group homes, volunteer social sponsors, and savvy school counselors—all these can keep improvement going strong for the long term.

These then are some "Head Gears" that can help set the stage for understanding what comes next—the rehabilitation process itself.

ELEVEN

THE PROCESS OF REHABILITATION

"He will manage the cure best who has foreseen what is to happen from the present state of matters."

—Hippocrates

The highway divider is looming in front of you, faster and faster, circling around as you go. You didn't see the dark oil spill on the road; it was slippery. You started to skid and you couldn't stop. And now, your car is spinning around, the divider closer, the sharp sounds of a car out of control augmented by your screams. No time to think, to realize that your car has spun out of control, that the impact has flung you forward, that your head has hit the windshield, crumbling the glass into a thousand shards. You have blacked out, blank and unfocused, a crumbled doll half out of the window of your car.

Your next conscious thought takes place on a hospital stretcher. The curtains are drawn on one side of the stretcher; the other is opened to allow these strangers, these white-coated strangers, to peer at you, poke you, stare into your eyes with a strange apparatus. Your thought is a cliché, but you don't realize that at first, you, who used to have such a fine sense of humor. Where am I? you think. You panic and try to push these strangers away. You grow more and more agitated; you pull at the restraints that are keeping you on the exam table.

You don't realize it yet, but you are in a nearby

neurotrauma center. A passing state police cruiser had seen your car seconds after it had hit the highway divider. He had immediately called an ambulance. But you know none of this. You lost consciousness for half an hour.

You will survive. You have a moderate closed head injury; you bruised your frontal lobes. You will need time to heal and for rehabilitation, motivation and patience to relearn the skills you have lost, determination to relearn motor coordination, love and support to help fill in the empty pockets of memory. You will need the knowledge and expertise of many rehabilitation specialists, including a neuropsychiatrist, someone who understands intimately the complex network of your brain, someone who will help you become aware of your deficits, who will help you learn how to accept them—and, most importantly, accept the new person who was born when your head hit the windshield...

This is not a scene from *Unsolved Mysteries*. Nor is it a Friday afternoon cliffhanger from your favorite soap. It is a scenario that occurs thousands of times every year. It's called traumatic brain injury—but its outcome can only be helped by rehabilitation.

We now know how the brain works. We have a working understanding of traumatic brain injury and its cognitive, physical, and psychosocial consequences. It is now time to turn to hope, to returning, to rehabilitation—the process of re-entry into the world.

RESCUE 911

My dramatic scene is more common than you might think. Most head injuries occur from car accidents, as well as motorcycle crashes, on the job falls, and muggings. Its victims may or may not be conscious when the ambulance is called and they are often rushed to a neurotrauma center for examination and evaluation.

It is there, at the center, that the initial treatment process is begun. The trauma team performs diagnostic tests, including CT scans and skull X-rays, to see what areas of the brain have been damaged and to what extent bleeding has occurred. (See Chapter 5 for more detail on diagnostic testing.)

It is also at the center where most life-threatening, critical medical problems, such as bleeding into the brain, are evaluated and treated. And, if the patient is in coma, it is classified according to the Glasgow Coma Scale (see Chapter 10).

BRAIN STORMING

Today's New Emergency Rooms

Hospital emergency rooms are fine for cuts, bruises, and more serious medical problems involving heart attacks and bleeding. But many standard emergency rooms are not equipped to handle severe head injuries. A traumatic brain injury requires specialized—and immediate—attention, the kind of care usually better provided at a modern neurotrauma center. Here, a trained staff, including neurosurgeons, respiratory therapists, and specialized nurses observe, evaluate, and treat possible internal bleeding, respiratory problems, increasing pressure within the head, and more. In fact, neurotrauma centers are so crucial in successfully treating head injuries today that when an accident involving TBI occurs, victims will often be flown by helicopter to the nearest one.

From the trauma center emergency room, the patient is transferred to the intensive care unit—where close monitoring of his condition continues until the most life-threatening problems from trauma are resolved.

Once his life is no longer threatened, the patient will be transferred to a general neurosurgical ward, where his continuing recovery will generally follow the steady progression through unconsciousness (or coma), disorientation, confusion, and possible amnesia to the time when he can once again remember things. With memory returning, more active rehabilitative efforts can begin, such as helping a person walk, dress, and wash himself again.

Divided into eight stages, this recovery progression is often described via the *Levels of Cognitive Functioning* developed by California's Rancho Los Amigos Hospital. As adapted from *The Nature of Head Injury* by Thomas Kay and Muriel Lezak, these eight stages are:

1. *No response*. The patient is in a deep true coma.
2. *Generalized response*. The patient sometimes responds to stimuli, but it is irratic; there is no pattern.
3. *Localized response*. The patient occasionally responds to specific stimuli.
4. *Confused-agitated*. The patient is very active, but he is unable to understand or process any information.
5. *Confused, inappropriate, non-agitated*. The patient consistently responds to simple commands, but continues to be fragmented; he cannot understand more complex commands or think on his own.
6. *Confused-appropriate*. The patient is exhibiting goal-directed behavior—but only when he's given an explanation of what he's to do.
7. *Automatic-appropriate*. The patient is able to go about his daily routine in the hospital and at home. But he does so in a robot-like manner; he has difficulty recalling what he has just been doing.
8. *Purposeful and appropriate*. The patient is alert. He knows what he's doing and why he's doing it. His past and present memories are well-integrated. He is a full-functioning member of society.

These levels are useful when describing a patient's functioning as he emerges from coma. Medical practitioners can circumvent lengthy explanations by declaring a patient at Level 6—or Level 5–6 (which would mean that his stage of recovery is in-between two levels and that he shows a combination of both levels' characteristics). Many rehabilitation centers also use a range of these levels as a criterion for admission.

But these levels are not black and white—and they should not be applied as such. They are primarily used in communication and in grouping patients for rehabilitative programs.

Each patient will go through these levels in his own time. Obviously, the longer the coma, the longer it will take him to get to Level 8—if he gets there at all. He will stay at the acute care hospital only until he is *physically* out of danger—which has nothing to do with his reaching a higher cognitive functioning level. At that time, he will be discharged—either to his home or, in most cases, to a rehabilitation center.

REHAB SAVVY

Ideally, rehabilitation will start in the intensive care unit of the hospital. In individuals with severe head injuries, most of the physical progress will usually occur between the time a patient emerges from coma and the following twenty-four months. For this reason, it's crucial to begin rehabilitation as soon as possible. In some circumstances, the neurotrauma center will notify us when a head injury patient comes in to its emergency room.

BRAIN STORMING

Proper diagnosis has five goals. To determine:
1. The presence of brain injury
2. The extent and the nature of any deficits
3. The role these deficits will play in the survivor's life—at home, on the job, and in social activities
4. The extent to which these deficits produce handicaps for the individual in his own world
5. An appropriate treatment program to minimize the impact of the handicaps on the patient's community and vocational re-entry.

Once it appears that there will be no more surprises from the initial brain trauma, a patient may be transferred to a hospital like ours—where, although physical progress is still evaluated and treated, behavior and cognitive rehabilitation take center stage.

The patient may be confused. She may be extremely agitated. She may have no understanding of where or who she is. It doesn't matter. Neurobehavioral rehabilitation can take place. This does not mean vocational retraining, such as learning to perform a new job. This type of rehabil-

itation must take a back seat when, in the case of severely
agitated patients, the need for physical safety is required.
But, even in these cases, activities of daily living (ADL),
can still be retaught—despite a patient's behavioral dyscontrol.

He might learn to control his explosive outbursts so
that he can feed himself. She might learn to shower despite
her confusion. He might learn to get from his bed to his
wheelchair by himself. Here's an example:

I have a 13-year-old patient at the Neurobehavioral
Institute of Houston who was thrown from an all terrain
vehicle. The girl had initially been brought to a Texas
hospital's neurotrauma center where she was diagnosed as
severely brain-injured. After two weeks of close observation
and diagnosis, she was transferred to a general rehabilitation hospital. However, she was so combative and hostile
that the staff was unable to manage her—and she was sent
to us.

This girl, whom I will call Mary, is still very confused
and agitated. She aggressively lashes out at our staff; she
screams and bites. She has remained incontinent and child-
like. Obviously, Mary would not do well in a group therapy
session. Nor would she sit with me when I first attempted
to talk to her. No, it's more basic than that. In addition to
supervising her medication and physical health, our inter-
disciplinary team and I spend hours every day teaching her
to go to the bathroom, to take a shower, to comb her hair.
Although she is still in the early stages of recovery, she can
begin to relearn basic human functions. Step by step,
through repetition and simple commands, my staff and I
are helping Mary recover. Think of it: if she doesn't learn
how to go to use the toilet independently now, right after
her injury, she might never learn. Because she is only 13
years old, this might mean 60 or 70 years of complete
dependency! Even if her extensive brain injury makes more
advanced rehabilitation an impossibility, Mary will still
function as a human being. She already knows how to turn
the water on in her shower, to regulate it, and pick up her
washcloth without assistance.

As Mary's example shows, it's never too early to start
rehabilitation. Although moderate or severely brain-injured
patients might be automatically transferred to a rehabilitation center, mildly brain-injured people are usually

discharged home. Unfortunately, we have seen the results that can occur in such a situation—from the teenaged bicycle rider who didn't get help for weeks to A.T., the advertising executive who became an alcoholic before she received help. And there is always the problem of "concussive" syndrome—with its psychological underpinnings that will undermine the mildly brain-injured person's life.

In short, most brain-injured people need some kind of rehabilitation—if not as an actual patient in a center, then on a daily or weekly outpatient basis.

And America is beginning to recognize this need. Not only has the 1990's been dubbed "The Decade of the Brain," but more than 500 rehabilitation centers dealing with head injuries have cropped up across the country—including those, like our Neurobehavioral Institute, which are even more specialized than the average rehabilitation center because they can offer real hope to those patients with post-acute behavioral problems. Many of these centers, including ours, have case managers who work with the families of brain-injured patients, guiding them through the emotional turmoil of the accident as well as the financial mazes of insurance and helping them understand the rehabilitation process itself.

Chances are, you are not now in a rehabilitation center's admission's office. In fact, you are probably sitting in your living room or lying in bed before turning off the lights. So, allow me be your case manager. Allow me to take you through the rehabilitation process your loved one might be about to begin—or is already involved in. Using the Neurobehavioral Institute of Houston as a prototype, I will briefly explain the techniques we use to compensate for cognitive deficits, develop appropriate behavior, and enhance self-awareness, the ways and wherefores of helping a brain-injured person re-enter the world. Let's begin.

THE PHYSICAL ENVIRONMENT

A good post-acute rehabilitation center has a "prosthetic environment." This means that everything is tailor-made for the handicapped person. From metal bars in the bathroom to wheelchair access doors and corridors, the center is designed to help compensate for any handicaps a brain-injured patient might have. This way, he won't have his handicaps accentuated.

At the Neurobehavioral Institute of Houston, we have four separate units. One is a closed ward, where severely brain-injured patients live and where some of our patients begin their recovery. Here, safety and security is primary. All the patients' rooms have doors for privacy, but they also have windows so that nurses and other medical staff can check in and make sure everything is okay—without disturbing them. These patients also have a kitchen and den area designed to help them relearn to cook their own meals—and clean up.

The other, open wards permit more freedom. Patients can walk or wheel themselves around the hospital; they do their own laundry, and make their own beds. They can go to the hospital cafeteria for their meals. Here, they will participate in therapy and retraining sessions as well as support groups—all of which helps them prepare for the outside world.

Because the environment is a prosthetic one, our patients can feel safe. They can work on their deficits without the additional stress of misunderstanding, rejection, or miscommunication they are not yet strong enough to confront in their own worlds.

PSYCHOPHARMACOLOGY

It's true. Drugs are not a panacea. Alone, they won't "cure" a brain-injured person. But nor are they "evil" elixirs that turn people into zombies—a myth that has stayed alive thanks to old Hollywood movies. Advances in biophysiology, in brain research, and in psychopharmacology itself have shown that certain medications can help a patient's chronic head pain. They can regulate her moods. They can calm his agitation. They can help prevent her seizures. Here are a few of the most common medications used in brain-injury rehabilitation:

1. Antidepressants

As we have seen, depression is extremely common in head injured patients. Sometimes a patient can become so depressed that it interferes with his rehabilitation. He might become suicidal as well. For these patients, an antidepressant, carefully supervised, can help. Antidepressants help restabilize the brain's natural homeostasis—restoring balance to damaged neuronal pathways. Because brain injury can cause an unusually high sensitivity to antidepressants, lower dosages are often successful in treating the problem without producing significant adverse effects. However, patients must be watched for any unusual side effects, including confusion and excessive sedation. Some brand names include: Norpramin, Pamelor, and Prozac.

BRAIN STORMING

The Good News About Brain-Injury and Depression

Brain injury no longer must exclude the benefits of antidepressants because of their side-effects. A relatively new antidepressant called fluoxetine has been found to work on the serotonin imbalance in the brain (a neurotransmitter believed to be involved in depression)—*but without the same side-effects as other antidepressants in brain-injured patients*. In a study I performed at the Neurobehavioral Institute of Houston, the only drawback in 50 percent of the patients was some sedation. And in two-thirds of the treatment group, their moods were substantially elevated.

Its brand name is Prozac.

---

2. Benzodiazepines (BZ)

These are anti-anxiety drugs usually used in emergency situations to help a brain-injured person deal with his agitation. Again, like the antidepressants, they must be closely monitored. BZs can also lead to disinhibition and, therefore, these drugs should only be given in cases of extreme anxiety and anger. Side-effects can include amnesia, excess sedation, and possible addiction. Some brand names include: Valium, Xanax, Ativan, and Librium.

3. Neuroleptics

These are the drugs primarily used for psychotic episodes. They are used for major breaks with reality and for hallucinatory behavior. In brain-injured patients, they have been found to curb excessive aggression. Unfortunately, they have many side-effects, including lowering the threshold for possible seizures, over-sedation, and Parkinsonian tremors. They should be used with caution, and only when rage and psychosis are at dangerous levels or when hallucinations interfere with a patient's functioning. Some brand names include: Trilafon, Navane, Prolixin, and Haldol.

4. Betablockers (BBs)

These drugs can work in both the peripheral and the central nervous system, "blocking" the symptoms of anxiety, including rapid heartbeat, high blood pressure, and stage fright. They have been shown to be successful in treating uncontrollable aggression in brain-injured patients—often without the extreme side-effects of neuroleptics. Some of the brand names include: Inderal and Visken.

5. Lithium Carbonate

Long the drug of choice for mood swings, lithium carbonate is actually a natural salt. It has been found to quiet the agitation brain-injured patients feel and stabilize their moods. It can also induce confusion, nausea, tremors, and apathy. Therefore, its use should be closely monitored. Brand names include Lithane and Eskalith.

6. Anticonvulsants

Yes, these drugs can help stop the seizures that affect many brain-injured patients, but they can also help improve aggression even in the absence of a seizure disorder. Newer agents such as Tegretol and Depakene, are preferred over older ones, such as phenobarbitol or Dilantin, because they may produce fewer cognitive side effects. Recently, physicians have been re-evaluating the need to treat all TBI survivors with anticonvulsants, preferring to use them only in individuals at high risk of having seizures or in those who have already had one.

* * *

Because these medications need to be closely supervised, initiating pharmacotherapy often works best within the prosthetic environment of a hospital. It's also important to keep in mind that in brain-injured patients, drugs are more likely to produce side effects at low doses. They also take more time to produce their optimum effect. Further, a physician should not prescribe any medication until a detailed medical history is taken and a complete neurological exam has been completed.

COGNITIVE REMEDIATION

It sounds serious—and it is. Helping brain-injured people redevelop their intellectual skills is one of rehabilitation's greatest challenges. As we have seen, head injuries often result in frontal and temporal lobe damage—where our abilities to think, to plan, to remember, to emote, and to gain insight and self-awareness are presumed to be located. However, it is not completely hopeless. Depending on the extent of the injury, degrees of cognitive capabilities can return over time.

One approach rehabilitation centers use in cognitive skill training comes from the research of Dr. Yehuda Ben-Yishay, who believes the goal of cognitive remediation is to help a brain-injured person function independently and appropriately in the community.

In his work at New York University, Dr. Ben-Yishay and his colleagues focus on three areas that need intervention in order to meet a brain-injured person's goal of achieving increased independence. They are:

- Personal hygiene and an ability to consistently carry out a daily routine
- Satisfying vocational pursuits
- Social adjustment and the ability to form relationships

To this end, he and his colleagues have developed a cognitive remediation program that has four basic principles which make it work:

Principle #1

A thorough neuropsychological exam must be performed to determine which areas of the brain are still functioning within normal ranges and which are impaired. However, this is easier said than done. Our current diagnostic tools are not always able to determine microscopic areas of damage. But knowing which areas of the brain are in working order can help a cognitive therapist immeasurably. He can actually use these working areas to help compensate for the areas that are impaired.

Here's an example: Say a brain-injured person still had his nonverbal recent memory intact, but his verbal recent memory abilities were impaired. A cognitive retraining therapist would concentrate on using his nonverbal memory to compensate for his deficient verbal abilities. In other words, a patient can be taught to write down things to remember in what we call a memory notebook rather than rely on his recent verbal memory recall.

Principle #2

Full advantage should be made of those processes that are intact—teaching problem-solving skills through them. In this way, a cognitive therapist can help a patient compensate for a deficit by utilizing residual strengths. For example, if a patient has difficulty with speech, a picture can be used to make his needs known to a therapist. He simply has to point to the picture of what he wants.

Further, in most brain-injured patients, there are still working neurotransmitters. In some circumstances, neurons have been damaged, but not destroyed. With time, their normal functioning may return. And, even if certain passageways are destroyed beyond repair, some studies have found that cognitive remediation can teach brain-injured people to "rethink," to use other, undamaged pathways to do the job.

Principle #3

Teaching the brain-injured is not like Mrs. Smith at the blackboard, looking at the students' raised hands or giving a spot quiz. Teaching is much more specific, with each task broken down into its component steps. Each step in problem-solving becomes linked to the next in an exacting chain of commands that will ultimately create a functional task. The emphasis is on procedural learning—and it works. A patient is trained by going over and over the basic, important tasks he'd once done automatically. The end goal is a relearned, functional, meaningful task. For instance, George, a young adult at the Neurobehavioral Institute, has intact writing and reading skills—but his recent memory is as swiftly gone as the wind. To help him function, he carries a large red notebook in which he writes down his schedule for the day—as well as detailed instructions for specific tasks. Let's say he is planning to dress himself this morning. His notebook would read:

MORNING DRESS PROGRAM

1. Go to dresser.
2. Open top dresser drawer.
3. Remove undershirt.
4. Remove underpants.
5. Remove socks.
6. Place underpants, undershirt and socks on bed.
7. Close top dresser drawer.
8. Open second dresser drawer.
9. Remove shirt.
10. Place shirt on the bed.
11. Close second dresser drawer...

And so on, each step completely delineated, one after another. In time, this task would become a part of George's procedural memory and, hopefully, he will no longer need to have each step written out for him. He will only need to be cued.

But even if George was incapable of condensing the steps for his morning dressing program, he could always refer to his notebook to both perform the task and see how it relates to the other activities in his day. His notebook allows him to be more independent.

Principle #4

This last principle in some ways is the most important. Not only must the intact areas of the brain be utilized, not only must a task be broken down to its smallest detail, not only must teaching be done in a repetitious manner—but all this must be done with patience and understanding. A good therapist will explain things over and over again—as long as it takes. She will provide valuable feedback. She will be positive and compliment a task well done.

A cognitive therapist will also work with language and speech therapists for a complete "remediation" package.

RE-ESTABLISHING THE SELF

But without self-awareness, none of these principles will work. People can't learn in a vacuum; they must be aware of what they are doing—and why. In addition to these four principles, cognitive remediation also involves therapy to re-establish self-awareness. As one study of 45 severely head-injured patients showed, those patients who were aware of their disabilities performed better in their tasks.

But teaching this awareness is easier said than done. Traditional one-on-one therapy is not likely to work with a brain-injured individual. Because this person has lost the ability to be self-reflective, she won't know what needs to be changed. A therapist can't ask her to describe her life or her problems; she might not be able to remember the content of one session to the next. Instead, a therapist must use paradigmatically oriented therapy, a basic, nonreflective therapy that has been successfully used in a number of post-acute rehabilitation programs. In paradigmatically oriented therapy, a therapist will explain, point-blank, what has to be changed. He will teach the process of self-awareness through the step-by-step chain of command of the "Memory Book" that George, for example, has found so successful.

Another technique used in paradigmatically oriented therapy is "before" and "after" snapshots. It's a process I had a great deal of success with in my sessions with the Urban Cowgirl. I showed her a photo of what she looked like before her brain injury, in her plain Levis, plaid blouse, and sneakers; I then showed her a more recent photo, showing her what she looks like now—with her rhinestone vest and studs. I'd repeat: "Look at this before picture. This girl looks like her friends. Now look at this after picture. This girl looks differently dressed than those around her."

A therapist will also use the feedback of family and friends—as I have done countless times, always pointing out that the patient's perception of himself may not be the one others see. Patiently, over and over again, I'll explain: "You say you don't believe that your parents aren't seeing the same *you* as *you* are, but we have to understand that their perceptions are as valid as yours."

Paradigmatically oriented therapy takes a long time. A trusting, involved, and supportive relationship between doctor and patient doesn't occur overnight. Nor does the process of self-awareness. There is no epiphany, no words of "Eureka! You're right!" Instead, there is a very gradual understanding, a very gradual belief that she is different, that others perceive her as different. Then, and only then, will the journey towards acceptance of this new self—and mental health—begin.

BEHAVIOR TRAINING

A study of 35 brain-injured patients at a head trauma rehabilitation unit found a great deal of success. Eight-five percent of them were discharged home. They were independent. They could perform their own "activities of daily living" successfully. They did not require special nursing or medical care more than every three months. But...they did have problems re-entering the world. They had difficulties on the job, at school, with their friends, and with their money.

Thus, "holistic" style of treatment is desperately needed for patients to successfully re-enter their former lives. It is a process in which every area of skill training works with the other. Cognitive training works with paradigmatically oriented therapy. Speech therapy complements behavioral training.

In this treatment model, understanding appropriate behavior is as important as solving problems. To truly become a functioning member of society, a brain-injured individual must learn how to live with others. And, as an added plus, behavioral training further promotes self-awareness.

But before appropriate behavior can be taught, inappropriate behavior must be stopped. Aggression, violence, promiscuity—these first must be addressed. Psychopharmacology coupled with consistent behavioral therapies often helps set the stage for successful neurobehavioral rehabilitation.

Behavioral training has a simple premise: A patient is "rewarded" when she acts appropriately, either with a positive social reward, like attention or praise, or with a tangible one—such as a token or points on a "point card." These "rewards" reinforce improved behavior.

To fully understand training, think of the famous management phrase: "Catching people doing it right." Inappropriate behavior is not usually criticized. Instead a reward isn't given out—or the negative action is ignored. In some circumstances, a token is given out after a patient has had fifteen minutes of controlled behavior. The more fifteen minute intervals of controlled behavior, the more tokens. The more tokens, the more privileges and rewards.

But, if the patient had, say, been verbally abusive to a peer during those fifteen minutes, the token would not be forthcoming—and neither would subsequent rewards.

Consequently, negative behavior *never* gets reinforced—and a patient never gets the attention he has been demanding in an inappropriate way. However, positive behavior is constantly being reinforced—at least every fifteen minutes. Thus, more appropriate behaviors are gradually shaped.

Behavior training is an ongoing process within the rehabilitation center. From keeping her physical therapy appointment to taking a shower in the morning, from attending a support group on alcohol abuse to making her bed—all these activities show appropriate behavior. And, at the same time, they move the retraining process forward.

In fact, behavior training includes a wide-ranging smorgasbord of services to help a brain-injured patient:

An *occupational therapist* might help him relearn how to appropriately feed himself, including everything from how to use a knife and fork to preparing a simple meal in a microwave oven.

A *social worker* will help the brain-injured patient determine personal, but realistic, goals and objectives to further develop planning skills—and hope for the future.

At the Neurobehavioral Institute of Houston, one patient's personal goals were:

1. Go back to work.
2. Be more active.
3. Get more therapy if needed upon discharge.
4. Work on marriage.

His objectives were:

1. Attend all groups and therapies.
2. Begin vocational evaluation.
3. Meet with my social worker and my wife for family therapy on Wednesday.

These statements were written out and tacked up on the patient's bedroom door as a daily reminder and a daily reinforcement: "You can do it. You can try. It's not impossible."

A *recreational therapist* might take the patient out to the supermarket where she can use the knowledge she learned in a finance/budget session. Here, she will buy food, pay for it, and count her change—all things she will need to do on her own.

A *group support session* might discuss the potential problems of alcohol and drug abuse following rehabilitation; they also provide helpful feedback, especially from peers.

Daily meetings with the staff and other patients help everyone air their issues; patients also get a chance to learn how to communicate with others. When the patients at the Neurobehavioral Institute of Houston wanted a washer and dryer to do their own laundry rather than send it back to their families, they brought it up at one of these meetings. The result? They received their appliances—and they also learned a valuable lesson in communication and self-reliance.

A *vocational therapist* might help her recognize her strengths and weaknesses as they relate to work. Or, as we do at the Neurobehavioral Institute of Houston, the vocational therapist might place her in a supervised job trial

BRAIN STORMING

Group Support

This "real world" to which the survivor hopes to return some day is composed of groups—large groups, small groups, quarters, triads, and pairs. Individuals are linked together as classmates, business partners, team players, families, partners in marriage or business, sellers, buyers, lovers, and friends. In the "real world," no one functions wholly in isolation; there are always others present, if only in a person's memories, thoughts, plans, fears, desires, and hopes. In a therapeutic environment, isolation is an unacceptable condition, except for brief periods as part of a behavior-modification program. Each brain-injured individual must interact regularly with at least one other person, or no change in his or her situation will occur.

(From "Traumatic Brain Injury and the Rehabilitation Process: A Psychiatric Perspective" by Irwin W. Pollack, in *Neuropsychological Treatment After Brain Injury*, Edited by David W. Ellis and Anne-Lise Christensen. Norwell, MA: Kluwer Academic Publishers, 1989.)

within the hospital itself—such as in the purchasing department helping with inventory.

Art and music therapists encourage a brain-injured patient's self-expression, helping him discover new avenues of communication that can help reduce inner tension and fill time in a productive way.

And, in fact, relaxation *is* crucial. A case study written up by Dr. Philip Barry in "A Psychological Perspective of Acute Brain Injury Rehabilitation," tells of a certain Mr. G who became extremely upset whenever he was faced with his language dysfunction. His speech therapist could get nowhere with him—until he was taught a deep-breathing, relaxation exercise. He would do this exercise before each speech session and, although his capacity to relax was limited due to his injury, he was eventually able to separate his anxiety from his language dysfunction—and to address each one separately. Relaxation helped Mr. G's speech therapy. His improved speech in turn helped his confidence. In other words, Mr. G was beginning to learn how to live independently and confidently in his new world.

This, in brief, is the rehabilitation process at work. But there is one more area that has not yet been addressed, an area that is as critical as any other to help a brain-injured person's re-entry into the community. It's called the family circle—and it matters a great deal. In fact, "family matters" need a chapter all of its own.

TWELVE

FAMILY MATTERS

"My family treats me like a baby."

—Brian, age 32, at the Neurobehavioral Institute of Houston

- Joe had finally been discharged from the hospital. He was able to function in the "real world." Although he was left with some behavioral and cognitive deficits, he was equipped with the tools to deal with them. But once he got home, all he did was sit in front of the television set. He refused to use his cane and go for a walk. He refused to sit down at the table to eat. He refused to join in any conversations. Joe had become the quintessential "couch potato...."
- Linda was sweet and unassuming when she returned home from the hospital. There was only one problem: she never stopped eating. Breakfast, lunch and dinner weren't enough. She was always at the refrigerator or at the kitchen table. Even late at night, she would eat chocolate bars, staring into the dark. She kept growing bigger and bigger.
- Joan was having a lot of trouble with her husband. She had listened to the case manager at the rehabilitation center. She had participated in individual and family therapy. She had even joined a support group. But she still couldn't cope. Whatever she said, wherever she went, Joe would be at her. "Why

110

did you say that?" "Who are you sneaking around
with behind my back?" "You wish I had died, don't
you?" "Admit it, you're plotting to have me committed...."

- Alfred loved Margaret. They'd been married for twenty
years and their time together just kept getting better and better. Now, at last, their kids were out of
the house, living lives of their own. Now, at last,
they can retire and take that leisurely cruise. Alfred
could turn one of the kids' rooms into a study; he
could write the novel he'd always wanted to write.
But all these dreams turned into so much smoke
when Margaret got into her car accident. One year
later and she's back home. But she's not Margaret.
She's another child. Alfred's feeling resentful, even
angry. He's afraid that his love is turning to hate.
The guilt is just about killing him.

Yes, a brain-injured person is often a tragic victim.
Frequently as a result of a split-second accident, he has lost
some of his intellectual capabilities. He has difficulties
controlling his behavior. And, above all, he has lost the self
he'd always been.

And what's also true is that a brain-injured person
needs loving care. One study found that the lack of a close,
sharing relationship made brain-injured patients suscepti-
ble to later emotional disorders. But there is something
else that study after study has discovered—or rather someone else.

It's called the family—and they need help, too.

THE TIES THAT BIND

Husband. Wife. Sibling. Child. There is nothing more powerful than family ties. In fact, as a whole, families strive to
maintain a "homeostasis," a balance between members
that keeps things safe and secure. There is an instinctual
family "hierarchy" in which everyone—from the cranky
breadwinner and the nurturing caretaker to the spoiled
brat and the voice of reason—has a role. This hierarchy is
dynamic; it changes as families age, as siblings are born
and grow up. But, generally, despite temporary setbacks

such as a problem adolescent, balance is restored. In fact, this need for homeostasis exists on a basic, primitive level; a shake-up in a family's balance threatens its continuation, its survival power. It is the reason why so many families deny, say, a teen's drug habit, why they become nervous when, say, a caretaker mom decides to get a job.

But when a family member becomes brain injured, this homeostasis is irrevocably ripped apart. In her book *On Death and Dying*, psychiatrist Elisabeth Kubler-Ross outlined six stages of grief a terminal patient goes through before coming to terms with his or her own death. They are:

1. *Denial:* "This isn't really happening to me."
2. *Anger:* "It's not fair! Why me!"
3. *Bargaining:* "God, if you just bring back my health, I'll be a good person forever."
4. *Depression.* "I hate this cruel world."
5. *Acceptance.* "So be it."
6. *Hope.* "Perhaps it's for the best. I leave a legacy of love."

As you can see, these stages of grief can be used for any traumatic event—be it death, divorce, or even the loss of a job. But studies have found that families of brain-injured patients do not go through these steps in sequence. What makes their families even more troubled is that they go through these in a more cyclical manner, in what Drs. Muir and Haffey call "mobile mourning." There is no finality, no death, no moving on. Instead, there are events, an ebb and flow of struggle. Prognoses change throughout the rehabilitation process; what starts out as a life-and-death emergency becomes an arduous waiting game through physical, cognitive, and behavioral rehabilitation—a game in which the rules change as the patient begins vocational training, as he comes home from the rehab center, as he re-enters the community. It is an ongoing process; these six stages occur dynamically—sometimes even at the same time. A family will move from denial to depression, hope to denial, acceptance to depression—depending on the current situation. In terms of psychological health, being in a family with a brain-damaged member is cause for stress with a capital "S."

THE "S" FACTOR

Stress can erode the best of families. Studies bear this out. Close relatives of 54 closed head injured patients were interviewed at 1 month, 6 months, and 12 months to see if their feelings of stress were at all alleviated. The answer was no. Although stress was extremely high at the time of the accident, it was still present six months and at one year. Another study of 55 relatives of severely brain-injured adults echoed these results. Interviews conducted at 3 months, 6 months, and 12 months found no difference in the relatives' stress levels: they remained constant—and high. The interviews also revealed that *emotional problems*, poor memory, depression and behavioral changes were the causes for the stress—not any physical impairment the brain-injured survivors might have had.

Yet another questionnaire, distributed mainly to mothers of brain-injured children, found that the biggest concern was what would happen to their sons and daughters if something happened to them.

More sobering news: a study of the wives of severely brain-injured soldiers found that stress *increased* after the one year mark. It was at that time that these wives realized that their husbands were not going to get better; their hopes for a miracle finally vanished. Depression ran high.

But, despite the high degree of pressure-filled stress, of emotional distress, and pain within the family sphere, home—believe it or not—is still where the heart is.

HOME SWEET HOME

No one likes to stay in a hospital indefinitely. There is nothing like familiar surroundings to make you feel better—and help create a feeling of normalcy. Traumatic brain-injured patients are no exception. But the only way to make that journey home a reality is through the involvement of the rest of the family.

But, this family involvement doesn't happen overnight. Nor does it begin the day the patient is discharged home. Since all of us would want to return home and have our lives as normal as possible, every effort must be made to encourage family involvement from the earliest stages of rehabilitation. Doctors, nurses, and case managers should all be accessible to family members. And, in turn, the family members themselves should be educated through support groups at the hospital and within one-on-one therapy sessions with a neuropsychiatrist or psychotherapist.

The goal is to help create a new balanced whole, a new homeostasis of familial give and take. And the only way for families with a brain-injured member to achieve this new "normalcy" is through education and self-insight—begun as soon after the accident as possible.

EDUCATION STARTS AT HOME

The sheets are clean, ready to be tucked in. The room is aired and ready. Your heart is filled with joy and love for the spouse or child who had been so close to death, who is, at last, ready to come home. Unfortunately, a brief "honeymoon" period at home is usually followed by a cold dose of reality. To prevent undue heartache, you need to know what to expect when you bring your brain-injured loved one home. Here, in brief, are a few of the "mind games" that you might be forced to play. In other words, problems that may crop up—and how to deal with them.

Mind Game #1: Temper Tantrums

Yes, when you take care of a brain-injured loved one, you'll come across a lot of these. Why the physical expression of their frustration and anger? Three reasons:

1. Difficulty putting needs into words
2. Lack of impulse control
3. Inability to cope with their environment and situation

Temper tantrums can begin and end abruptly—and with absolutely no provocation. One minute, your wife might scream: "I hate your guts!" An hour later, she might smile at you and wonder why you're upset.

Winning strategies: Whenever possible, ignore them—and don't remind your spouse about them later. Chances are, she will have forgotten she'd lost her temper. Try to redirect her focus to something more positive.

Mind Game #2: Egocentrism

After a brain-injury, many people become extremely self-centered, reverting back to the days when they were mere tots. It's not their fault. Sympathy towards others, empathy, a larger world view—none of these are possible without insight. And lack of insight, as we have discovered, is a common cognitive deficit. In his mind, the world truly revolves around himself.

Egocentrism is not exactly an endearing trait. And, unfortunately, it can make family members back off even more from their loved one—and, in turn, make him even more self-centered.

Winning strategies: Do not give in all the time. Don't allow him to believe that every one of his demands will always be met—immediately. If possible, try to get him to join a local head injury support group. And join one yourself; it will help you cope.

Mind Game #3: Emotional Lability

A loss of control over one's emotions is a frightening prospect to anyone; unless we are in dire pain or in the depths of a dark depression, we usually can keep our emotions in check—at least in public. But a brain-injured person may lose this capability. He doesn't know when to stop—or where. Mood swings are usually quick, erratic, and frequent. She can't stop crying. He gets tears in his eyes when he watches television commercials. She giggles before she speaks. He starts crying whenever the past is brought up.

Winning strategies: Address the behavior—not the feelings behind the tears. Ask him to "calm down." Tell her to "Go to her room for a bit to calm down." Try to keep the home environment as stress-free as possible.

Mind Game #4: Denial

No one wants to face a difficult reality—especially when it means facing a "new self" with cognitive and behavioral deficits. If he doesn't have to examine himself, he won't have to believe that he can no longer fly a plane. If she doesn't take a hard look at herself, she won't have to face the fact that she can no longer take care of the kids.

Unfortunately, denial will sabotage any rehabilitation—at home and at the hospital. After all, if someone doesn't believe he has problems, why does he need therapy?

Denial can also be dangerous. He might attempt to use a chainsaw—and not be at all concerned about safety. She might try to drive to a doctor's appointment—and get hopelessly lost.

Winning strategies: If something your loved one wants to do isn't dangerous—go ahead and let him. It will encourage his independence. But do be around to supervise. If denial continues for any length of time, enlist the help of a therapist or contact your local rehabilitation center. It's crucial for both of you.

Mind Games #5: Depression

We have seen how common depression is in brain-injured individuals. Your loved one could be depressed if he exhibits:

1. A lack of motivation, particularly in the morning.
2. Excessive sleeping or waking up too early in the morning.
3. An inability to enjoy anything and everything.
4. Withdrawal and passivity.
5. A habit of watching much too much television.
6. Loss of appetite.
7. Unexplained episodes of crying.

Winning strategies: Seek professional help—to avoid even more tragedy. And, remember, *his depression is not your fault*. Keep your own guilt and depression at bay with your own individual therapy.

Mind Game #6: Obsession

No, you are not caught in a real-life *Fatal Attraction*. Obsessive-compulsive disorders occur in brain-injured people because of memory loss, anxiety, and neurological damage. He might forget that he'd already mentioned his aspirin twenty-five times in the last hour. She just can't stop talking about her brain injury; she has no control over her need to wash her hands over and over again. He obsesses about his old job, literally talking about it for hours. She hoards old newspapers and other trash in her room.

Winning strategies: Yes, this type of behavior will try anyone's patience, but don't confront it head-on. This will only lead to *more* obsessing—this time about you. Try to redirect him to a new topic. And, because this behavior has a lot to do with anxiety, attempt to reassure him; praise her progress.

Mind Game #7: Dependency

It's true that your loved one will be more dependent on you. But dependency is a relative term. You might have to remind him every night to brush his teeth; you might have to stand there with him while he does his nightly routine. You might not want your impulsive, brain-injured daughter going out by herself—for fear she might come home pregnant.

Neither of these two situations are dependency problems. Educating a person with memory loss or taking precautions with someone who lacks impulse control is a case of common sense. Here are some examples of real dependent behavior—pure and simple:

She might want you to make all her phone calls. He might want you to stay in the room with him until he falls asleep. She won't let you go out of the house—unless you take her with you....

Winning Strategies: Don't isolate yourself from others. Have friends and other family members come to the house. Take your loved one to a support group where he can make new friends.

These are only a few of the problems you and your injured loved one might face. For further help and advice, contact your rehabilitation center. Its staff is there to help both of you.

BEFORE YOU START....

Here's some sensible, reassuring advice you need to hear before you can begin to take care of someone you love, before you can begin your home rehabilitation program. As adapted from Dr. Muriel D. Lezak's article, "Living with the Characterologically Altered Brain Injured Patient" that appeared in *The Journal of Clinical Psychiatry*, they are:

1. Anger, frustration, sorrow, and guilt are natural feelings.

It's difficult enough having the responsibility of taking care of someone you love—without being weighed down with guilt. Think of it: your spouse or your child has been cranky, irritable; he hasn't ever voiced his thanks—or love, for that matter. In fact, he hasn't been the same since his accident. Why wouldn't you be angry or sad—and why wouldn't you, at times, wish he had died in the accident.

BRAIN STORMING

A Story of Hope

Her parents called her their "Miracle Child." She is Cindy Holley Sharif today, but ten years ago, she was simply Cindy Holley—a young college girl who'd been in a terrible car accident. She suffered severe head injuries; it would be a long road back. Cindy stayed in a coma for a week. Eventually, she entered rehabilitation. She became violent and foul-mouthed. "I felt like my youth and life had been robbed from me," Cindy told *Parade* reporter Claire Carter. She was also told that she might never walk again.

But time, perseverance, determination, and a strong will won out. Today Cindy can walk; she is no longer that violent person. She does have some residual impairments; she is blind in her right eye and she can't stop moving her foot. But she went back to college—and got all A's. She married and became a successful prison case worker. "I hope I would be an inspiration for someone else," Cindy told the *Parade* reporter. "I'm probably a better person for having gone through the accident. I'm much more together and brighter. It made me aware of an inner strength I didn't know I had."

Remember, words are not deeds. Wishes do not become reality.

2. Before you can take care of anyone else, you have to take care of yourself.

This sounds simple—but many spouses and parents who are taking care of brain-injured patients forget this. It's easy to slip into a "martyr" role, never finding the time to, say, get your hair done or see a movie. After all, your child needs so much; your husband wants all of your attention. But duty is one thing—and your well-being is another. In fact, your first duty is to yourself—and your health. How can you possibly take care of anyone if you let yourself run down? How good a job do you think you'd do if you became sick, tired, or depressed? Indulge yourself once in a while. Get in some leisure time and exercise. And do this without a sense of guilt. Remember: by taking care of yourself, you're taking better care of your loved one—and everyone else in the family.

3. Trust your instincts.

Your spouse might be contrary. He might not want to take his medication. She might try to push you away when you offer a helping arm during a walk. And, if behavior is a real problem, he might even threaten you.

Don't try to handle this alone—nor should you comply with his outrageous demands. Call your doctor or case manager. Seek help. If living with a brain-damaged loved one is so pressure-filled and dangerous, it might be wise for you to consider alternatives. There are always choices—if you know where to look.

4. Get educated.

As with most things in life, knowledge is power. It can make the difference between a balanced home situation and one that begins to disintegrate before your eyes. Knowing what to expect from your brain-injured spouse or child with a TBI means knowing what to do about it—as well as possibly circumventing an uncomfortable situation completely.

Furthermore, don't forget that you too went through a

trauma—and you too need help. If it is your spouse who has been injured, you must deal with the role change that invariably takes place—from equal partner to dependent "child." If it is your child, you must make peace with the fact that the future envisioned for him might never happen. And whether husband, wife, child, or sibling, you must face the reality that the person you loved is changed; he or she has become a different person. It's important to seek out the advice and insights of a therapist to help you understand, accept, and decide what to do with this tragic situation. Take advantage of any support groups at a local rehabilitation center. Write to The National Head Injury Association at 333 Turnpike Road, Southboro, MA 01772. Or call their family helpline at 1-800-444-NHIF. They are there to help. You are not alone.

5. A hard reality: You can't do everything for your loved one—and you shouldn't feel guilty if he doesn't improve in your care.

Tough, but true. As we have seen, most of the rehabilitation progress occurs within the course of a year or two. But, although you might not help him regain all his cognitive skills or all his memory, you can make life comfortable for him. You can make peace with his new "self" and enjoy your time together—and your time apart.

Beginning a new life is never easy. But re-entering the family circle can be made easier for someone you love if you understand what you're up against—and what you can and can't do to help. Take advantage of community services; there are field trips, camps, and other support group activities for brain-injured people. Ask your rehabilitation center or vocational therapist for help in finding employers who are willing to hire brain-injured people. A study of brain-injured patients returning to work found that supportive employment intervention helped them find a job and keep it—becoming a valuable member of the company team.

In other words, all is not lost for you—or the person you love. Life with a brain-injured loved one is hard, but it doesn't have to be impossible.

Nor does it have to end in tragedy.

EPILOGUE

THE FUTURE IS WAITING

Recently, one of my brain-injured patients said to me: "I feel like I lost my future."

The only reasonable reply I could give him was, "Yes, that's true." But I added an important note: "You've definitely lost **one** future. But not **the** future. Together, we can shape a new future, one where you can still find meaning and purpose in life."

It took several months of almost daily "coaching," but eventually he got the message—and the hope it implied.

We have now gone over the miracle of the brain, how it works and what happens when it gets hurt. We have seen the tragic results of brain injury—and the myths we perpetuate to keep the reality of that tragedy at bay.

But we have also seen how denial only sabotages success. Physical handicaps, cognitive deficits, psychosocial problems: all of these can be treated and even if full "recovery" is not possible, a survivor can at least come to accept the remaining difficulties and continue on with life.

Acceptance of that "new" self is a vital component of successful brain injury rehabilitation. It has always been my goal as a neuropsychiatrist to help my patients embrace this new self—and to help the families of my patients, if not embrace, at least accept their loved one for who he or she is now.

As I mentioned within these pages, Congress has dubbed the 1990s, "The Decade of the Brain," and it is indeed cause for celebration. Inroads made in diagnostic technology, in pharmacologic therapy, in rehabilitation techniques, in head injury education—all hold hope for the future.

But hope is a fragile commodity. It must be carefully cultivated and constantly nurtured. Slow, but steady, progress is the hallmark of my work. But it is the courage of my patients and their families that keep me going. And it's also words like this, from that same patient I mentioned above: "We're still people. We still count. And, in spite of our problems, we can still live and be loved. We can still work and be productive. I may not have the same life I had before, but I can still have a life that matters."

Defeat?

Never.

I hope you find this same inspiration—and the same courage—to fight your own private war with brain injury. I hope this book will help you win some of its battles.

And, if nothing else, remember this: there are people out there, imperfect though they may be, who truly care. And there are others, like some of my patients who have shared their stories with you in this book, who continue to defy fate.

To defiance.

To life.

SOURCES

Barry, Philip, "A Psychological Perspective of Acute Brain Injury Rehabilitation," *Cognitive Rehabilitation* (July/August 1986), pp. 18–21.

Baker, Susan P.; R.A. Whittfield, and Brian O'Neill, "Geographic Variations in Mortality From Motor Vehicle Crashes," *New England Journal of Medicine*, 316:22 (May 28, 1987), p. 1384–7.

Ben-Yishay, Yehuda, and George P. Prigatano, "Chapter 27: Cognitive Remediation." *In: Rehabilitation of the Adult and Child with Traumatic Brain Injury*, edited by E. Griffith and M. Rosenthal. Philadelphia: F.A. Davis Company, 1990.

Blackerby, William F., III, "Head Injury Rehabilitation: Sexuality After TBI," *The HDI Professional Series on Traumatic Brain Injury, No. 10*. Houston, Texas: HDI Publishers, 1988.

Bond, Michael, "Chapter 8: The Psychiatry of Closed Head Injury." *In: Closed Head Injury: Psychological, Social, and Family Consequences*, edited by Neil Brooks. Oxford, England: Oxford University Press, 1984.

Bromberg, Walter, M.D., "Psychiatric Traumatology," *Psychiatric Annals*, 14:7 (July 1984), p. 500–505.

Brotherton, Frank A.; Linda L. Thomas; Ira E. Wisotzek, and Michael A. Milan, "Social Skills Training in the Rehabilitation of Patients with Traumatic Closed Head Injury," *Archives of Physical Medicine Rehabilitation*, vol. 69, October 1988, p. 827–832.

Calub, Connie; Dana S. DaBoskey; John Burton; Cathy Cook; Lis Lowe; Dorothy McHenry, and Karen Morin, and the staff of Tampa General Rehabilitation Center, Tampa, Florida, "Teaching the Head Injured: What to Expect," *The HDI Coping Series, No. 5*. Houston, Texas: HDI Publishers, 1989.

Campbell, Catherine Henry, "Needs of Relatives and Helpfulness of Support Groups in Severe Head Injury," *Rehabilitation Nursing*, 13:6 (November–December 1988), p. 320–326.

Carter, Claire, "She's Our Miracle Child," *Parade Magazine*, May 14, 1989.

Cassidy, John W., "Fluoxetine: A New Serotonergically Active Antidepressant," *Journal of Head Trauma Rehabilitation*, 4:2 (1989), p. 67–69.

"Pharmacologic Treatment of Post-Traumatic Behavioral Disorders: Aggression and Disorders of Mood." *In: Neurobehavioral Sequelae of Traumatic Brain Injury*. Ed. RLI Wood. New York: Taylor & Francis, 1990.

Chenier, Thomas C., and Leonard Evans, "Motorcyclist Fatalities and the Repeal of Mandatory Helmet Wearing Laws," *Accident Analysis and Prevention*, 19:2, 1987.

DeBoskey, Dana S.; Judy Beahon; Karen Morin; Robert Rosen; Bonnie
  Wells, and the staff of Tampa General Rehabilitation Center, *Actions
  and Reactions: A Stroke Manual for Families*. Houston, Texas: HDI
  Publishers, 1989.

——; Karen Morin, and the staff of Tampa General Rehabilitation
  Center, Tampa, Florida, "Head Injury: A Guide for Families," *The
  HDI Coping Series, No. 1*. Houston, Texas: HDI Publishers, 1989.

——; Connie J. Calub; John Burton; Karen Morin, and the staff of
  Tampa General Rehabilitation Center, Tampa, Florida, "Life After
  Head Injury: Who Am I?," *The HDI Coping Series, No. 4*. Houston,
  Texas: HDI Publishers, 1989.

Division of Epidemiology, New York State Department of Health, "Bicycle
  Safety," *Epidemiology Notes*, 3:5 (May 1988).

Do, Hyunok K.; Debra A. Sahagian; Lois C. Schuster, and Susan E.
  Sheridan, "Head Trauma Rehabilitation: Program Evaluation," *Rehabilitation Nursing*, 13:2 (March–April 1988), p. 71–75.

Dobkin, Bruce H., "Head Trauma," *New York Times Magazine*, October 9,
  1988, p. 50–1.

Dunn, William, "Soviet Scientists Studying Sakharov's Brain," *USA Today*,
  February 8, 1990.

Edwards, Patricia A., "Rehabilitation Outcomes in Children with Brain
  Injury," *Rehabilitation Nursing*, 12:3 (May–June 1987), p. 125–127.

Evans, Leonard, "The Fraction of Traffic Fatalities Attributable to Alcohol,"
  *Transportation Research Board, Paper No. 890374, 69th Annual Meet-
  ing*, Washington, D.C., January 7–11, 1990.

——, "Passive Compared to Active Approaches to Reducing Occupant
  Fatalities," *General Motors Research Publication GMR-6596*, March
  10, 1989.

Garoutte, Bill, and R.B. Aird, "Behavioral Effects of Head Injury," *Psychiatric Annals*, 14:7 (July 1984), p. 507–514.

Giles, Gordon Muir, and Jo Clark-Wilson, "The Use of Behavioral Techniques in Functional Skills Training After Severe Brain Injury,"
  American Journal of Occupational Therapy, 42:10, (October 1988), p.
  658–665.

Golden, Charles, "The Luria-Nebraska Neuropsychological Battery in
  Forensic Assessment of Head Injury," *Psychiatric Annals*, 14:7 (July
  1984), p. 532–538.

Goldstein, Kurt, "The Effect of Brain Damage on the Personality," *Psychiatry*, vol. 15:3 (1952), p. 245–260.

Haas, Janet F., D. Nathan Cope, and Karyl Hall, "Premorbid Preva-
  lence of Poor Academic Performance in Severe Head Injury,"
  Journal of Neurology, Neurosurgery, and Psychiatry, vol. 50 (1987),
  p. 52–56.

Halls, John R.; Hernan M. Reyes; Maria Horvat; Janet L. Meller, and
  Robert Stein, "The Mortality of Childhood Falls," *Journal of
  Trauma*, 29:9 (September 1989), p. 1273–1275.

Henderson, Victor W., "Outcome Prediction After Severe Closed
  Head Injury in Adults," *Bulletin of Clinical Neurosciences*, vol. 52
  (1987).

Hinds, Michael deCourcy, "Bareheaded Motorcyclists Pressed Anew to
  Cover Up," *New York Times*, January 14, 1989, p. 50.

Jacobs, Harvey E., "Chapter 20: Adult Community Integration," *In: Traumatic*

Brain Injury (Comprehensic Neurologic Rehabilitation) vol. 2, edited by P. Bachyrita. New York: Demos Publications, 1989.

———, "Chapter 12: Long-Term Family Intervention" Part III: Rehabilitation Techniques." *In: Neuropsychological Treatment After Brain Injury*, edited by David W. Ellis and Anne-Lise Christensen. Norwell, Mass.: Kluwer Academic Publishers, 1989.

Jackson, Howard F., "Finding the Self: Personality and Emotional Recovery Following Traumatic Brain Injury," presented at the fourth Annual Symposium on Advances in Head Injury Rehabilitation, Dallas, Texas, March 2–4, 1989.

Katz, Howard T., Testimony to the United States Senate Subcommittee on the Handicapped Recommending Solutions to Some of the Problems Encountered by Head Injured Survivors and Their Families, April 12, 1988.

Kay, Thomas, Ph.D., and Muriel Lezak, Ph.D., "Chapter 2: The Nature of Head (Injury)," *In:* Corthell (Ed.), *Traumatic Brain Injury and Vocational Rehabilitation*. Menomonie, WI: University of Wisconsin-Stout, 1990.

Kinsella, Glynda; Moran, Carmel; Bruce Ford, and Jennie Ponsford, "Emotional Disorder and its Assessment Within the Severe Head Injured Population," *Psychological Medicine*, vol. 18 (1988), p. 57–64.

Kwentus, Joseph A.; Robert P. Hart; Edward T. Peck, and Susan Kornstein, "Psychiatric Complications of Closed Head Trauma," *Psychosomatics*, 26:1 (January 1985), p. 8–17.

Lam, Chow S.; Brian T. McMahon; David A. Priddy, and Anne Gehred-Schultz, "Deficit Awareness and Treatment Performance Among Traumatic Head Injury Adults," *Brain Injury*, 2:3 (1988), p. 235–242.

Lehman, L.B., M.D., "Preventing and Anticipating Neurologic Injuries in Sports," *AFP*, 38:4 (October 1988), p. 181–184.

Levin, Harvey S., and Robert G. Grossman, "Behavioral Sequelae of Closed Head Injury: A Quantitative Study," *Archives of Neurology*, vol. 35 (November 1978), p. 720–727.

———, Arthur L. Benton, and Robert G. Grossman, *Neurobehavioral Consequences of Closed Head Injury*. New York: Oxford University Press, 1982.

Lezak, Muriel D., "Brain Damage is a Family Affair," *Journal of Clinical and Experimental Neuropsychology*, 10:3 (June 1988), p. 351–361.

———, "Living with the Characterologically Altered Brain Injured Patient," *Journal of Clinical Psychiatry*, 39:7 (July 1978), p. 592–596.

———, "The Problem of Assessing Executive Functions," *International Journal of Psychology*, vol. 17 (1982), p. 281–297.

Linge, Fredric R., "What Does It Feel Like To Be Brain Damaged?" *Canada's Mental Health*, Health and Welfare Canada. September 1980. p. 4.

Long, Charles J., and Thomas A. Novack, "Postconcussion Symptoms After Head Trauma: Interpretation and Treatment," *Southern Medical Journal*, 79:6 (June 1986), p. 728–732.

MacKenzie, Ellen J., Sam Shapiro, and John H. Siegel, "The Economic Impact of Traumatic Injuries: One-Year Treatment-Related Expenditures," *Journal of the American Medical Association*, 260:22 (December 9, 1988), p. 3290–3296.

McKinlay, W.W.; D.N. Brooks; M.R. Bond; D.P. Martinage, and M.M. Marshall, "The Short-Term Outcome of Severe Blunt Head Injury as Reported by Relatives of the Injured Persons," *Journal of Neurology, Neurosurgery, and Psychiatry*, 44:6 (June 1981), p. 527–533.

McMahon, Brian T., and Susan M. Flowers, "The High Cost of a Bump on the Head," *Business and Health*, vol. 3 (June 1986), p. 47–51.

McMordie, William R., and Susan L. Barker, "The Financial Trauma of Head Injury," *Brain Injury*, 2:4 (1988), p. 357–364.

Meeks, John E., *High Times Low Times: How to Cope with Teenage Depression*. New York: Berkley Books, 1989.

Oddy, Michael; Michael Humphrey, and David Uttley, "Stresses Upon the Relatives of Head-Injured Patients," *British Journal of Psychiatry*, vol. 133 (1978), p. 507–513.

Ornstein, Robert, and Richard F. Thompson, *The Amazing Brain*. Boston: Houghton Mifflin Company, 1986.

Pollack, Irwin W., "Chapter 5: Traumatic Brain Injury and the Rehabilitation Process: A Psychiatric Perspective. Part I: Theory and Intervention." *In: Neuropsychological Treatment After Brain Injury*, edited by David W. Ellis and Anne-Lise Christensen. Norwell, Mass.: Kluwer Academic Publishers, 1989.

Powers, John, "Risk Too Great," *Boston Globe*, March 9, 1990.

Prigatano, George P., "Work, Love, and Play After Brain Injury," *Bulletin of the Menninger Clinic*, vol. 53 (1989), p. 414–431.

Prigatano, George P., "Bring It Up in Milieu: Toward Effective Traumatic Brain Injury Rehabilitation Interaction," *Rehabilitation Psychology*, 34:2 (1989), p. 135–144.

Prigatano, George P., "Chapter 16: Psychiatric Aspects of Head Injury: Problem Areas and Suggested Guidelines for Research," *In: Neurobehavioral Recovery from Head Injury*, Harvey S. Levin, Jordan Grafman, and Howard Eisenberg, editors. Oxford University Press, New York 1987, p. 215–231.

Restak, Richard M., *The Brain*. New York: Bantam Books, 1984.

Rome, Howard P., Old Wine in New Bottles (re: "Reflections on Traumatology"), *Psychiatric Annals*, 14:7 (July 1984), p. 567.

Rosenbaum, Michael, and Theodore Najenson, "Changes in Life Patterns and Symptoms of Low Mood as Reported by Wives of Severely Brain-Injured Soldiers," *Journal of Consulting and Clinical Psychology*, 44:6 (1976), p. 881–888.

Rutherford, William H., Merrett, J.D., and McDonald, J.R., "Sequelae of Concussion Caused by Minor Head Injuries," *The Lancet*, January 1, 1977, p. 1–4.

Sacks, Oliver, *A Leg to Stand On*. New York: Harper & Row, 1984.

——, *Awakenings*. New York: E.P. Dutton, 1983.

——, *The Man Who Mistook His Wife for a Hat and Other Clinical Tales*, New York: Harper & Row, 1987.

Silver, Jonathan M.; Stuart C. Yudofsky, and Robert E. Hales, "Chapter 10: Neuropsychiatric Aspects of Traumatic Brain Injury." *In: The American Psychiatric Press Textbook of Neuropsychiatry*, edited by Robert E. Hales, and Stuart C. Yudofsky. Washington, D.C.: American Psychiatric Press, 1987.

Slaby, Andrew E., *Aftershock: Surviving the Delayed Effects of Trauma, Crisis and Loss*. New York: Villard Books, 1989.

Sosin, Daniel M.; Jeffrey J. Sacks, and Suzanne M. Smith, "Head Injury-Associated Deaths in the United States From 1979 to 1986," *Journal of the American Medical Association*, 262:16 (October 17, 1989), p. 2251–2255.

Thompson, Robert S.; Frederick P. Rivara, and Diane C. Thompson, "A Case-Control Study of the Effectiveness of Bicycle Safety Helmets," *New England Journal of Medicine*, 320:21 (May 25, 1989), p. 1361–1367.

Tyerman, Andrew, and Michael Humphrey, "Changes in Self-Concept Following Severe Head Injury," *International Journal of Rehabilitation Research*, 7:1 (1984), p. 11–23.

Vogenthaler, Donald R., "An Overview of Head Injury: Its Consequences and Rehabilitation," *Brain Injury*, 1:1 (1987), p. 113–127.

Walker, David E.; Virginia Blankenship, and Jeffrey A. Ditty, "Prediction of Recovery for Closed Head Injured Adults: An Evaluation of the MMPI, the Adaptive Behavior Scale, and a 'Quality of Life' Rating Scale," Braintree Hospital Eighth Annual Traumatic Head Injury Conference, October 14, 1987.

Ward, Christopher D., "Encephalitis Lethargica and the Development of Neuropsychiatry," *Psychiatric Clinics of North America*, 9:2 (June 1986), p. 215–224.

Wehman, Paul; Jeffrey Kreutzer; Wendy Wood; Henry Stonnington; Joel Diambra, and M.V. Morton, "Helping Traumatically Brain Injured Patients Return to Work With Supported Employment: Three Case Studies," *Archives of Physical Medicine and Rehabilitation*, vol. 70 (February 1989), p. 109–113.

Wesolowski, Michael, with Arnie Zencius, Richard J. Zawlocki, and William H. Burke, "Head Injury Rehabilitation: Developing Self Control," *HDI Professional Series on Traumatic Brain Injury, No. 14*. Houston, Texas: HDI Publishers, 1988.

———, "Head Injury Rehabilitation: Managing Anger and Aggression," *HDI Professional Series on Traumatic Brain Injury, No. 6*. Houston, Texas: HDI Publishers, 1988.

Wood, R.L., "Chapter 10: Behaviour Disorders Following Severe Brain Injury: Their Presentation and Psychological Management." *In: Closed Head Injury: Psychological, Social, and Family Consequences*, edited by Neil Brooks. Oxford, England: Oxford University Press, 1984.

INDEX